30-minute-a-day

BODY CHALLENGE

also by Simon Waterson:

Commando Workout: 4 Weeks to Total Fitness

30-minute-a-day

BODY CHALLENGE

Simon Waterson

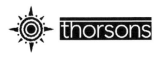

Thorsons
An Imprint of HarperCollins*Publishers*
77–85 Fulham Palace Road
Hammersmith, London W6 8JB

The website address is:
www.thorsonselement.com

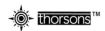

and *Thorsons* are trademarks of
HarperCollins*Publishers* Limited

First published 2003

10 9 8 7 6 5 4 3 2 1

A catalogue record for this book
is available from the British Library

Photography by Robin Matthews

ISBN 0 00 715607 3

Printed and bound in Great Britain by
Scotprint, Haddington, East Lothian

contents

preparing for the body challenge

Commandos are men and women who come from all areas of the military to go through the toughest fitness training known to man and then maintain peak mental and physical condition at all times. Since becoming a personal trainer I have adapted the basic physical and mental principles of this elite group to train ordinary men and women (as well as Bond stars and celebrities!) into extraordinary shape. This book is based on those principles, and is the fastest way there is to tone up and get fit. Do it and you'll not only reach your physical potential, but you'll discover new reserves of self-respect and determination. Prepare to take on the Body Challenge!

In the same way that commandos are self-selected, choosing to rise above their normal rank and go through intensive training to become the best, since you've picked up this book you are already sure to relate to the drive to be your best. This book will show you how.

This book is a combination of commando grit and celebrity chutzpah. You probably have your own celebrity idols – bodies that you admire, whether they're film stars or track stars. It might surprise you to learn that most of these bodies are created using bread and butter fitness exercises. Fads come and go but fitness basics like running, ab crunches and press-ups are here to stay, because they work efficiently and effectively.

During my training I learnt the motivational and training skills needed to keep myself in peak mental and physical shape at all times. Once you've graduated from the Body Challenge, you'll be equipped to do the same, and be able to maintain a high level of fitness in just 30 minutes a day, without a gym or any fancy equipment.

For the last eight years, I've applied the discipline and efficiency of the marines to personal training, working in the pop and film businesses with stars such as Geri Haliwell, Halle Berry and Pierce Brosnan. People imagine stars have hours a day to devote to getting fit, but in fact many train for a short time – very intensely. That is just what you are going to be doing on this program: getting into your best shape ever in just 30 minutes a day, 4 or 5 times a week.

With this program:

- You're in control of your fitness, it's not in control of you. This program is short, fast and effective – you can't let a fitness program monopolize your whole life.
- You will push yourself beyond the limits of your own expectations. This is a hardcore book for people who want hardcore results. It's not a fitness fad, but a program for life. Once you've mastered the techniques here, you can keep fit anywhere, at any age, with minimal equipment and time.
- You will learn how to manipulate yourself mentally to think you can do things that may initially seem impossible – and then you'll see the results!

- You will challenge yourself, be honest with yourself – and enjoy yourself! Don't be afraid to admit that you've got weaknesses, just learn how to improve on your strengths. Mastering fitness is very de-stressing.

Remember you don't have to do this program, no one is forcing you to – but if you make the choice it will have a big impact on your life. And you will earn respect, not only from family and friends, but most of all from yourself.

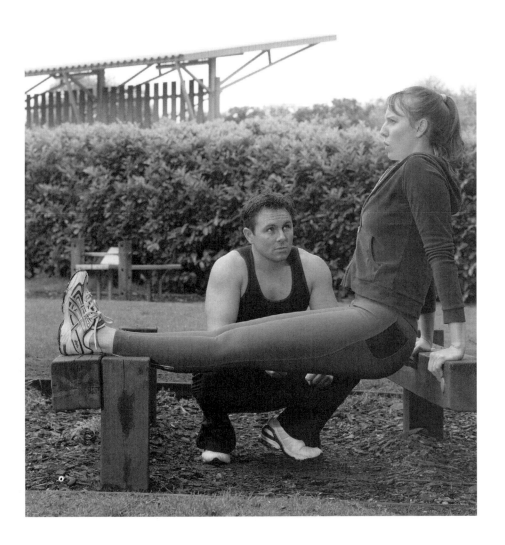

starting out

If you're under-fit and overweight, you're in the perfect place to begin.

This program will be easier if you have a base level of fitness, from doing some kind of fitness activity for 3–6 months (whether it's walking every day or working out a few times a week). If you have been a couch potato for the last year or so then enter into exercise very lightly! You can adjust this program to suit you, but you may want to improve your base fitness with four weeks of powerwalking and jogging before you start.

The programs here are appropriate for all sorts of fitness levels and body types, because you set your own intensity levels and learn how to adapt diet and weights, according to whether you want to burn fat or build muscle.

But play safe. See your doctor before you start if:

- You are overweight. Your doctor can check if you have heart or other problems that could be made worse by exercise.
- You have high blood pressure. Hypertension is the biggest cause of stroke and heart disease, but it usually shows no symptoms. Regular exercise is an effective way of lowering blood pressure, but it is essential you do it with medical supervision.
- You have an irregular heartbeat, or if your heart rate takes a long time to return to normal after physical exertion such as climbing stairs.
- You have a history of high cholesterol or any medical conditions that might affect your ability to do intense training.

Do you drag yourself out of bed every morning, and long to bounce out of bed instead?
The Body Challenge will give you energy to spare.

Do you dress to cover your physical shortcomings, rather than being able to wear anything?
The Body Challenge will give you your best body whatever your physical type: making you fitter, leaner, firmer and stronger. Geri Halliwell, Halle Berry and Pearce Brosnan all do the same basic training, but altering weights and repetitions according to whether they want to slim down, or muscle up.

Do you want to feel 'fit enough' – whether you're running after children, footballs or deadlines?
The Body Challenge will give you explosive power and stamina.

Do you want to be able to keep fit wherever you are?
The exercises in this book have been done for years and years. They work because they are high impact and efficient, using multiple body parts – and you can incorporate them into your every day life, wherever you are.

the 4-week concept

There are 7 different programs to work from in this book, and they are all designed to be done for 4 weeks at a time. When I worked with Halle Berry on *Die Another Day* we had just 4 weeks to get ready for that notorious bikini scene – and just 30 minutes a day. In the same way athletes have off-season and on-season training, in the film business there are off-screen and on-screen bodies, with actors and actresses taking 4–8 weeks to change their body image for roles.

Apply the same concept to yourself. Keep in good shape all year round, but use the 4-Week Concept for special things in life – whether it's toning up for a wedding, getting fit for a skiing holiday, slimming down for the beach or improving your fitness before the start of the soccer season.

the fastest way on earth to get fit

There has been a misconception for years that getting fit takes a long time. It doesn't. New research backs up what I have discovered already and confirmed in work with my clients – you can get a great body in just 30 minutes as long as you're working efficiently.

Normally the main bulk of a workout is done in 30 minutes, whether people are going to an exercise class or working out by themselves into the gym. This program just makes sure you can leave straight after that!

Intense training is hard but has its benefits. Not only will you lose weight, firm up and have better posture and digestion, you will feel mentally calmer, have more stamina and radiate confidence. And you'll have lots of time left to enjoy the knock-on effects of this on the rest of your life.

functional fitness

Even though we live in a world of technology where we are shuttled around in cars, trains and buses, we still need fitness for our everyday lives. If you only train on a treadmill or on weights machines your body will only be efficient at working out on those machines. That's why this program uses free weights and body weights to train. When you move freely and use your own bodyweight as resistance, you recruit your muscles to work together, improving strength, stability and balance into the bargain. You become 'functionally fit' and able to apply your physical strength, power and endurance to all situations. The result is a more balanced body – in terms of appearance and function – and a more efficient one.

Using fancy workout machines is a bit like doing trigonometry in maths – you can get very good at it, but how are you going to apply it to your everyday life? Separate yourself from the rest. Become physically and mentally stronger in life – resilience is a quality, like a muscle, that gets stronger with daily exercise.

true success stories

After my first book, *The Commando Workout*, I got e-mails from all over the world from people who had enjoyed the program. They came from all walks of life. The program was used by housewives in the Australian outback, rugby teams in South Africa and a hockey team in Canada. Some people who did the program were about to join the forces and did the program to improve their pre-military fitness. But it was also adopted by a Welsh swimmer for out-of-water training before the Commonwealth games, as well as a Colorado fire and police academy. Here's what some of them said:

Hi Simon and team

I'm a 28-year-old Australian female who stumbled across your book in a store and was so keen about what you had to say I went home and read the entire book overnight and I started the training the very next morning. I just finished the 4-week program and now have the willpower to continue this for the rest of my life. I want to thank you so much and when people ask how I got so slim I say, 'with my commando fitness trainer Simon' and I feel so ready to run through the bush with my backpack on I can achieve anything. THANK YOU

See ya mate

Kirsty

Dear Simon

Great book! I too am ex-army, and I am the Director of a Police academy and a Firefighter academy in Colorado. I am going to require all my students to buy your book to supplement their fitness portion of the training. I had literally dozens of fitness manuals to choose from before choosing yours but think yours will assist them in their outside training on their own time. I've been doing your program and found it very efficacious!

Professionally,

Mick, Colorado.

Hi there

I recently bought your book 'Commando Workout' and I would just like to say how impressed I have been. The results for me were instant. I noticed greater definition in my arms and legs overnight, and can really feel the extra muscle in my chest and shoulders … Great! I haven't lost a huge amount of weight yet, but I have noticed significant benefits in stamina, muscle definition and the overall good feeling that you get from exercise. I am very pleased. Thanks for coming up with such a challenging plan … I am so astounded that I cannot stop recommending it to my friends and colleagues!

Rodger, Saudi Arabia

Hi Simon and fit team
Congratulations on a fantastic book! I've nearly finished the program and have never felt fitter. Thank you. I am looking forward to your next one!
Nick, Australia

Hi Simon
My wife and I are half way through your program and despite the icy pavements in the mornings and freezing garage in the evening we're loving every minute of it. Huge thanks.
Al'n'Jax, Edinburgh, England

Hi Simon
Great book. Thoroughly enjoyed it and completed all sections religiously! Just completed my first Half Marathon in 1.40 with little stress. I am certainly really enjoying the benefits of increased fitness!
Regards,
Gregor, London

As you can see from these e-mails the program works for all sorts of people. Are you ready to start? If you have read the first book, this allows you to move on to something more advanced. But if you're a beginner you can start from scratch here. The two books work well together whichever one you do first.

key points

- You don't need to spend hours a day in a gym to get fit.

- Using this program you'll achieve much more than just weight loss.

- You'll get results whether you're male or female, fit or unfit.

- You'll learn skills you need to keep yourself in shape for the rest of your life.

the mental challenge

Everyone planning to do the Body Challenge will have something

standing in their way – work, stress, partners, bad habits. Don't

worry! Everyone will have their own personal obstacles and

learning how to get over – or under – them is part of the program.

Mental conditioning comes before physical conditioning, but by

adopting the commando philosophy: 'Improvise, Adapt and

Overcome' you'll see knock-on effects on your mind, body

and life.

Positive mental attitude is crucial to fitness. If you know how to control your brain, your body will be transformed – after all, it's your head that tells your body to stop, not the other way around! Once you've trained yourself mentally, physical training becomes a lot easier. You'll find it easier to work out when you want and how you want. Your head will push you beyond your limits – and you'll enjoy it.

Hundreds of people from all walks of life and from all over the world e-mailed me after my first book, from the super-fit to the super-unfit, to say how much they liked the program. And they all had two things in common. One, they said the program is really hard, but they liked the toughness of it. Two, they said they felt proud of themselves for completing it.

You can feel proud of yourself too. I didn't design this program to be easy, but in this book I have given you all the mental muscle you need to see it through. Mental conditioning comes before physical conditioning, and that's what this chapter is about – learning how to overcome obstacles, and stick to your goals when the going gets tough.

The commandos have a simple philosophy: improvise, adapt and overcome. It refers to everything they do: whether it's crossing a river, overcoming a mountain or completing fitness training in tough situations. If it was cold we'd warm up a bit longer, if it was scorching we'd drink more water, but whatever the circumstances we'd get the workout done. Your goal while you're signed up to this program is just that: improvise, adapt and overcome – and get the workout done.

be prepared

You will change mentally and physically doing this program. You'll become mentally more efficient and physically more alert – not just when you're exercising, but also when you're working and socializing. Your concentration span will increase and your productivity in life and work will go up – in the Far East, workers in some finance houses start the day with 30 minutes of group fitness to maximize productivity!

But as you set off on your journey, there are two obstacles that you can guarantee you will meet on the way – so be prepared!

obstacle 1 – expect unexpected resistance from hostile quarters

Everyone will be happy to see you making changes in your life, right? Wrong. Other people are the biggest obstacle you will come across in this program. You may encounter a certain amount of jealousy, and you may find other people feel threatened by you changing. Friends and family may feel left out of your new regime, annoyed they don't fit into your new eating and drinking habits, or fearful that they are not changing with you. Save all your energy for the program by only telling the people who you think are going to have a positive influence on you.

sssh! developing social fitness awareness

What goes around comes around, so don't be nasty to people less fit than you. In the same way that some celebrities make a point never to be nasty to people on their way up, in case they meet them on the way down, you need to practise good fitness karma. Right now you're focused, but you haven't always been, so be aware of how you talk about your regime in a social situation – don't brag, or big yourself up. Avoid talking about it with people who aren't as disciplined as you, or who would love to be on a program, only they haven't yet got to the stage where they can make the commitment. And don't try and convince others that your program is the only one to do. Everyone is unique, and by demeaning other programs to make yourself feel better, you'll only end up tripping yourself up. Tell a select few who will encourage you but won't judge you, otherwise it often pays to keep quiet.

obstacle 2 – things never go quite according to plan

However polished your plan, the reality is always slightly different. And it is the same with getting fit. You'll surprise yourself in what you can and can't do, you'll encounter tiredness and muscle soreness you're not accustomed to, and you'll run into difficulties you couldn't anticipate. Know this up front and it'll be a lot easier to maintain a positive mental attitude.

It's also worth preparing yourself for the fact the Body Challenge is hard. How hard? Hard enough to make changes – on a scale of 1–10 this is between 7 and 10 in terms of difficulty. The Body Challenge caters to all levels of fitness – some people will be doing 2 press-ups a minute in the circuits, others will do 20 – but everyone in the program will find it difficult. But everything that you experience as part of that difficulty will help you become mentally and physically stronger.

TIP: A positive mental attitude is the key to success. Project forward not back – forget what you could do 5 years ago, think about what you can do today. Keep in the moment and go with the flow.

To ensure that you succeed with anything in life, mental preparation is vital to make your progress as smooth and easy as possible. By eliminating all the hurdles that you can before you actually embark on the Body Challenge will help you to achieve your goals with the least difficulty. And always concentrate on the positive aspects of your performance and resist dwelling on the past or comparing yourself with how much you were able to do before. Focus on what you are going to do for yourself – right now, this minute, today!

step 1: making it to your workout – 10 ways to make sure you never miss a workout

Most people intend to work out more than they do, but things get in the way. The only difference between the fit and unfit person is that the fit person has tactics to deal with distractions. Here are my top 10 ways to make sure you never miss a workout again:

1. schedule your workout

Arrange your week like a campaign. At the beginning of the week, put your workout times into your diary (use the weekly planners at the end of the book). If you can exercise at the same time each day, all the better: having a familiar routine increases your chances of sticking with it.

2. be prepared

If you work out in the morning, lay out your kit the night before so you can step straight into your trainers when you get up. If you work out after work, pack your gym bag before bed. You'll save time and be more likely to stick to your plan.

(Prepare for workouts when away from home too: with a pair of trainers and set of dumbbells you can do these workouts almost anywhere.)

3. be trustworthy

Afford yourself the same respect you afford other people. Once you've made appointments: keep them.

4. praise yourself

When you work out tell yourself that you're doing well, and other encouraging words that will boost you. Think 'Right now everyone else is sat on their bottoms watching the telly and I'm doing this' and feel proud. Positive self-talk is a psychological enhancer, boosting your mental strength.

5. pick a time you like

You may have heard morning workouts are better, since you can burn off more fat after an overnight fast, or that they help you build more muscle because testosterone levels are higher.

Don't worry about things like this. The optimal time for you to work out is when you can. Get stuck in first, and address the fine details of optimum workout times when you become more efficient.

6. cross your workout off

Do your workout, then cross it off. Research has found that exercisers who keep track of workouts make more progress than those who don't.

7. stick with your program

Resist switching from program to program or adapting your workouts – it can undermine results. Make a commitment to stick at the same program for 4, 8 or 12 weeks and you will see maximum return for your efforts.

8. measure results

Choose a benchmark on which to measure your increasing fitness. This program allows you to choose one of a number of goals, such as losing fat, building muscle or getting fitter for a particular sport.

When you've chosen your goal (see Chapter 7, 'The Workouts'), measure progress towards it. Then if your waistband is becoming looser or your biceps are becoming stronger, you'll know the program is working.

If you are working towards becoming leaner, buy some scales that measure body-fat percentage so you can see your body composition change over the weeks.

9. clean up

Personal presentation is as important as fitness – it is part of the healthy body–healthy mind synergy. When you're clean it is one less distraction – dirt can make you feel uncomfortable.

When you're doing this program, look after yourself. Floss your teeth, wear clean gym kit, change your workout socks; it will make you feel fitter and more alert. And when you finish your workout, shower straight afterwards – it signifies the end of the hard arduous workout, and the beginning of your office day or evening, feeling fresh and exhilarated inside and out. Grubby kit won't get you fit.

10. plan your meals

Many people skip their workouts because however much their mind is telling them to workout, their body is telling them to eat, because they're starving. Plan your meals and snacks so you never have to workout when your energy is flagging (*see* Chapter 4, 'The Body Challenge Eating Plan').

Even with all the above 10 tactics in place, you'll still get caught short now and then – by a late office meeting, a birthday party you'd forgotten about, or an emergency at home. If the hurdle's important (and it has to be important – not just an Indian meal down at the local!) then remember the motto: *improvise, adapt and overcome.* Can you do part of your workout? Can you do something else instead – walk briskly to and from the party, or do an abs circuit while you wait for the plumber? If you can't, don't beat yourself up, and don't panic. We all have to have a social life – it's OK once in a while to relax, rest and reschedule. Remember you're in control of your fitness, it's not in control of you. Show your mental strength.

step 2: making every workout is a great workout – 5 mental tricks to make every workout great

Once you've put on your trainers, you have another challenge: making the most of your workout time. The more single-minded focus you can apply to your workouts, the greater the results will be.

Some days your body will be keen for the challenge. Other days it'll be a struggle to get your workout done. On days like these you need a few mental tricks up your sleeve in order to find that little bit extra you need to give it your all. Here are some tricks I use with clients.

1. just start

Some days you'll feel like you can't be bothered. Make a pact with yourself: 'If a workout is in my diary, I'll start. However much I don't feel like doing it, I'll get into my trainers, and into the gym, and begin.'

The chances are that once you're there, you'll feel you might as well do the work-out – after all it's just 30 minutes.

2. use reverse psychology

If you challenge yourself with a little reverse psychology, you'll be surprised what you can do. Say, 'Today I'm going to use a heavier set of weights, I know I'll never do it, but I'll give it a go.' Or, 'I'll never beat yesterday's number of reps, but I'll try.' I use this kind of reverse psychology on my clients all the time. People nearly always rise to the challenge, and they nearly always win.

3. use carrots

You are doing a great thing, sticking to this program, so treat yourself well. Motivate yourself by using carrots whenever you can. Say, 'If I complete this week's workouts I'll know it's time to buy a really great bikini for my holiday.' Or, 'After I finish this circuit I'll cook myself my favourite meal tonight.' Reward yourself for your accomplishments.

4. find your 5th gear

This program is the fastest way there is to get fit. But it's also one of the hardest. To see the results you need to find your fifth gear. When the going gets tough, dig your heels in. Be determined. Separate yourself from the rest – everyone else is in 4th gear, pull away in 5th.

We normally saunter through life doing a bit of this and a bit of that. When you feel like flaking out, remember: the extra 3 reps add up, the extra 100 calories a day add up, the extra workouts add up. And what they equal is a better body.

5. remember difficult days are part of the program

Some days are harder than others. One day you'll be sprinting around the park, the next day your legs may feel so heavy it's hard to keep going. This doesn't mean you should take an extra rest day or forget the program – feeling stiff and tired are part of getting fitter. After a hard workout, the immediate effect is that your body feels weak. But after a few days it will recover and be stronger than it was before. Keep your effort level constant, follow the diet rules so you are properly nourished – and stick with it.

working out with a buddy

If you can, find someone to train with so you can benefit from teamwork. Research shows that exercising with someone else improves adherence and motivation – knowing your friend is waiting at the park gates at 7.30 am makes you that much more likely to be there on time.

A buddy can also make you feel good – challenge and praise each other, be motivating, send text messages to give each other a boost if you're down.

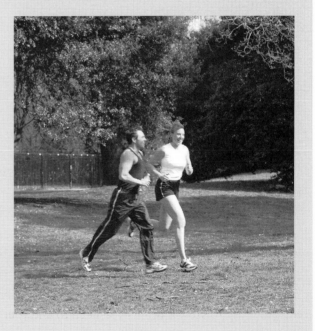

dealing with stress

A lot of stress is self-induced, and while you can massage the tension out of your body, you can't massage your brain. But you can learn how to channel stress into energy and productivity. Find something that releases it for you and turns a negative into a positive. This could be contemplation, meditation, action or – even better – exercise. Exercise can take you out of your day, release tension and aggression, and burn off adrenalin. Learn how to channel negative stress into a fitness positive.

step 3: motivating yourself all year round – 7 reasons to workout even when you don't feel like it

This program is designed to be done for 4, 8 or 12 weeks at a time. After that I suggest doing something different for a month or so to challenge your body in a different way, as variety keeps the mind and body alert. However, for most people the issue is not whether they can follow the same program for 12 months of the year, but whether they will exercise at all for months at a time!

This is unfortunate because maintaining a balance is better than going from one extreme to another. Regular exercise is one of the easiest ways to turn yourself into a happier, healthier, more productive person all year round. New Year gyms are full of people with fresh ambitions and before summer most of us get ready for baring our bodies. But wouldn't it be better if your body was permanently ready to get into your beachwear? If you didn't go through a see-saw cycle of loss and gain?

The secret of a good body all year round is enjoying what regular exercise gives you on a daily basis, rather than doing it so you feel better two months down the line. If every session makes you feel better about yourself, then you'll always go. Here are my top 7 reasons for exercising. Think about them and during the cold, dark months when you're wearing three sweaters and you'll still find that you want to go to the gym.

1. raise your metabolism

Exercise builds muscle mass and this raises your resting metabolism – meaning that you burn more calories even as you sleep. Plus, just 30 minutes of strength training elevates the metabolism for up to 48 hours (the fitter you are, and the more lean muscle tissue you have, the longer the afterburn effect lasts). And the higher your metabolism, the easier it is to keep weight off.

2. get happy

My clients find exercise distracts them and takes them out of their day, and they often leave sessions refreshed, energized and re-motivated to do other things in life. Whether you're at the gym or in the park, it is good to be mentally absorbed in something other than work.

Research also shows that strength training reduces tension, depression and anger, and that even 20-minute workouts trigger an enhanced mood that will last for several hours. And if you're happy when you've finished your workout and go into a social environment, this will rub off onto other people as well.

3. detox

Modern life is toxic – convenience foods, pollution, alcohol, smoking (passive or otherwise) and coffee all bombard the body with harmful substances that can make you feel lethargic. Exercise helps you sweat them out, and keeps your body working efficiently so you feel healthy and energetic.

Plus, as people become fitter, they start detoxing their life without realizing it – what was 20 cigarettes becomes fewer, what was 3 expresso coffees becomes 2 bottles of water. That's your mental strength and stamina working subconsciously. As you get fitter, your body starts to crave things that are good for you. But be patient – it takes 6 weeks to change what your taste buds crave for.

4. improve your thinking power

Research shows that exercise can help people be more creative. Working out will help you come up with solutions to problems, increase productivity, and improve your whole brain capacity. It unlocks different areas of the brain, helping you to come up with new ideas.

5. increase your financial fitness

Workout for a payout? It could happen. In the Far East workers do 30-minute workouts before the start of the day – together, as a company – to help improve productivity and efficiency. As an individual you'll find that the focus, energy and drive that regular exercise gives you can help your bank balance.

6. boost your immune system

Want to avoid the colds and sniffles that half your office falls prey to? Then exercise! Studies have found that aerobic exercise raises the immune system's ability to recognize bacteria and viruses – and thus fight them off. Researchers in North Carolina have found that people who exercise regularly (in this case, by walking) had half the number of colds and sore throats in a 12-week period than those who were less active.

7. raise your self-esteem

All of us can benefit from higher self-esteem. Working out regularly is like giving yourself a self-worth certificate – it makes you feel good about yourself and helps you feel important to society and other individuals. Keep a check so you can see yourself improve, and then receive an extra boost to your self-esteem when you reach your target!

step 4: knowing when to work out – and when not to

By now you'll be getting the idea that there are very few reasons not to work out. But what if you're ill or hung over? Here's my guide:

DO: Work out on a hangover – but with lots of liquid. Hangover equals dehydration equals workouts that feel harder. When your body is dehydrated, it can't carry as much oxygen, so making you feel tired – but this is no reason to quit! Hangovers are self-induced – now it's time to self-induce exercise!

Counteract your hangover by drinking lots of water throughout the day, and have an isotonic sports drink half an hour before you work out to help you rehydrate. Eat foods that will help balance your blood sugar and regain energy, and choose things that have a placebo effect on you – some people find beans on toast makes them feel better, for others it's fresh juice.

DON'T: Work out if you're ill. This doesn't mean that you should skip a session whenever you have a slight sniffle: ill means not being well enough to go to work, or suffering from a heavy cold or flu. If your symptoms are below the neck – coughing, aching muscles, nausea, wheezing – then take the day off. If they're above the neck – runny nose, sore throat, headache – it's OK to workout if you feel up to it. Do the first 10 minutes on half power, and if you feel better, carry on.

DO: Work out if you're menstruating. Women's strength varies throughout the month and many women find workouts feel harder just before their period. However it's well-known that exercise can help even out hormonal fluctuations, mood swings and reduce period pain. Work out on half power for the first few days of your period if you like, but keep to your plan.

DON'T: Work out on an injury. You can't exercise through joint pain – you'll simply make it worse, and if you exercise on an injury, something that could take a few days to heal may take a few months. The chapter on injuries deals with this in more depth (*see* Chapter 3, 'How to Prevent and Recover from Physical Injury'). But the general rule is that if you have knee, shin, ankle or back pain, then see a physio and get yourself better before you carry on. If you are out of action for a couple of weeks you will need to start at the beginning of the program again – don't fret about this, though, because you'll be starting from a higher level of knowledge and fitness than before. If your injury was only for 2 or 3 days, then if you feel confident enough you can restart from where you left off.

DO: Workout if you're stiff. You will recover faster from a harder workout if you use the same muscles lightly the following day, as it gets blood and nutrients to muscles and helps them repair. DOMS (Delayed Onset Muscle Soreness) is a natural product of increasing fitness, and occurs when small muscle fibres are ripped during exercise, then repairing themselves to become stronger and more efficient. This program takes DOMS into account by giving you rest days and working out on alternate parts of the body, so stiffness is no reason to skip a session. Neither is it something to aim for – don't get addicted to getting sore. After the first few weeks you'll find you don't have to hurt to make progress.

key points

- Be positive: whatever obstacles stand in the way, you can overcome them.

- Be prepared: the more you think ahead and plan your workouts the more likely you are to complete them.

- Be proud: keep a detailed log of the training you've completed to track your progress.

how to prevent and recover from physical injury

Millions of men and women throughout the world suffer from some kind of sports injury. The more you know about injuries, the quicker you can get back in shape. This chapter will help you identify the difference between a training strain and a more serious injury. It will also help you prevent injuries, and recover from them if they do occur. We are all prone to the odd ache and pain but if you learn about your body you'll know which ones to grin and bear, and which ones not to dismiss.

Taking the right course of action after an injury can make all the difference between being out of action for a short and a long while. It can also affect how prone you are to injuries in the future – many injuries happen for a reason, whether it's poor technique or an underlying muscle imbalance. Play detective when you experience aches and pains and you may drastically reduce your chance of injuries recurring. This is important, as studies of injuries experienced by footballers have shown that the severity of second or third injuries (re-injuries) is greater than initial injuries.

This chapter is designed to help you avoid making common mistakes, help you look after your body, and advise you when an injury needs expert treatment. Studies have found that the more involved people are in sports and exercise, the more depressed and anxious they become when they do get injured. I've found that knowing how to look after yourself better, and take an active part in rehabilitation, is one of the best ways to counteract feeling blue when you're injured.

hitting the ground running

For some people, just carrying their own bodyweight can put extra stress and strain on the joints and cause a lot of problems for knees, ankles and backs. This doesn't mean you should stop exercising – far from it. If you want an active old age then exercise is the best way to ensure that you have it, but it does mean you need to pay attention to what is going on in your body.

Common knee, shin and ankle injuries are due to muscle imbalance and there are various ways of correcting them, from rest and rehabilitative exercises to a pair of orthotics (sports insoles that change the position of the foot and thus change walking and running style).

Exercising on injuries can make them worse, and even cause permanent damage, so here's how to keep on running without problems. The golden rules:

- **Pay attention to pain**. It's a sign that something is wrong. This may be down to wrong trainers, wrong technique or something that will take a little longer to fix – muscle imbalance or overuse – but never ignore joint pain, as it is always telling you something.

- **Take rest days**. Sometimes pain may be the result of too much activity with not enough rest – physios see a lot of pain that comes from lifting too much weight in the gym, or running at the same intensity for too long. The programs in this book have been particularly geared to prevent this, so make sure to take rest when it's due.

twisted ankles

Twisted ankles are rarely the disaster you might imagine. Most people can get back in training within a few days. However, it is also the injury most likely to recur – once ligaments in the ankle are stretched they rarely return to their previous length, and you are more likely to twist them again. Be preventative: find out what is going on, and try to correct it.

the injury

Most sprains are outwards, when you roll on the outer part of your foot and sprain the weaker ligaments on the outside of the joint. A forward sprain can occur during kicking, and has also been seen in climbers when force is placed on the front of the ankle, tearing the tendons. Twisted ankles are common football injuries but could happen to you on this program if you're running or powerwalking outdoors.

the solution

1 RICE. Follow the instructions (*see* box below) as soon as you can after going over on your ankle. The faster you get your ankle in a compression bandage and ice, the better.
2 Take it easy for 3 days – after which time you should see an improvement. During this time you can carry on with the Body Challenge as long as you avoid certain activities. Don't run or powerwalk. Do go swimming. Hold on to the side of the pool and move the ankle through its range of movement in the water (toes up, toes down and ankle circles). Static recumbent cycling (on a gym bike where you sit with back supported and legs extended in front of you) is also fine for twisted ankles, as long as you push predominately with the good leg and ensure the injured ankle stays in its normal position

in the pedal. In the days following injury, both these activities will keep the ankle moving which will help the joint retain elasticity, and prevent the Achilles tendon and the tendon at the front of the ankle from stiffening (which will mean it takes longer to heal).

3 Get some support. When exercises and activities can be performed without pain, start back on low-intensity programs to allow the body and injured area to adapt. Consider using some form of taping or bracing, or wearing a neoprene ankle support in the short term. The support should only be used for as long as you feel you *really* need it. Don't use it all the time, or your muscles won't be encouraged to take the strain and regain strength. As a guide, simple injuries to the side of the ankle usually involve wearing some form of ankle protection for 4–6 weeks post injury whilst training or playing sport. Taper the use of it during this period, gradually doing more activity without support.

4 Do rehab exercises. One sprained ankle often means many sprained ankles if you don't correct the underlying weakness in the joint. Sports physios use balance trainers to strengthen the ankle and avoid future injuries, and these are now readily available to the public. (*See* box on page 28, 'Strengthening the Ankle'.)

5 Consider consulting a physio. If within 3–4 days the symptoms have not improved, or if they have worsened with symptoms such as increased swelling, then consult a physiotherapist who will assess any associated damage to ligaments and tendons, and treat the ankle with methods such as deep tissue massage and manual manipulation.

the 'rice' drill

RICE – which stands for Rest, Ice, Compression and Elevation – is the pinnacle of self-care for many injuries. Here's how it works:

REST – avoid contracting injured muscles through exercise for a few days after injury, or as long as it takes for internal bleeding and inflammation to calm down. This helps them heal faster.

ICE – apply ice to an injured muscle as soon as possible to reduce inflammation, so blood and nutrients can get to the injured part and repair it. The easiest way to apply ice is to wrap a bag of frozen vegetables in a towel against the injured area, or you can buy reusable gel packs specifically for this purpose. Apply ice for 15 minutes every 1–2 hours for up to a day. More is not always better in the ice department, the idea is to take down the swelling not freeze the life out of the tissue!

COMPRESSION – apply a firm bandage against the affected area to reduce internal bleeding and minimize any swelling. Compression should be carried out both during and after ice, and the bandage width should be related to the affected area. The bandage should be pressed to the area firmly but not so hard as to cause pain.

ELEVATION – use a sling for upper limb injuries and rest lower limbs on a chair or a pile of pillows. Position the arm so the wrist is up and the elbow is above the heart, or the legs above the pelvis. Elevating the limb encourages blood to flow away from the injury and back towards the heart, thus it is crucial that the lower limb is above the pelvis.

The first 24 hours after injury is the best time to use RICE – and the time to avoid the following: heat, heat rubs, hot baths, alcohol, moderate/intense activity, massage.

strengthening the ankle

To train the small muscles (proprioceptors) that automatically stabilize joints, practise balancing on one leg. Use a wobble board or mini trampoline to strengthen stabilizing muscles further. Sports physios use these to train micro-muscles and torn ligaments – just improvize balances and workout moves and the act of staying upright will do the work. Or have someone throw balls to you to improve your reactive balance.

Other good exercises for ankles: step-ups and running in a figure of eight. Reebok Core classes take place on a wobble board, based on the rehabilitative boards used by physios. These are ideal for people with weak ankles.

painful knees

Knees are a common area to feel pain. Don't despair! Knee pain is actually very useful in that it can alert you to biomechanical problems in your make-up that may otherwise go undetected. Knowing about them means you can do something about them – and avoid problems later in life. What you do depends on what kind of pain it is.

the injury – anterior knee pain or runner's knee

The most common type of knee pain is commonly called runner's knee, a dull occasional pain behind the knee cap. There are two causes of this the first being a sudden dramatic increase in workload. The knee is not a very stable joint, and relies on leg muscles around the knee to support it adequately. If you have just started a new program and experience pain, then it could be that you're not used to what you're doing and need to reduce the workload and then increase it again more gradually. As a guide, marathoners follow a 10% training rule – never increasing the intensity of training by more than 10% a week – that's 10% faster, 10% longer, or 5% of both. Bear this in mind if you're new to exercise.

The second cause of anterior knee pain is the kneecap being out of alignment, so instead of bones gliding over each other, they wear away the cartilage that cushions them, so they grate. This tends to be the kind of mild nagging recurring pain that few people do anything about, but you should! You are only born with a certain amount of cartilage on the end of your joints, and once this is gone, that's it forever. Take preventative action now to avoid problems in later life. Slight twinges may be an indication that in 5 years time you'll have a problem that's more serious.

the solution

1 Take a week off high impact work and lower body work (less than a week if less pain is felt). Continue doing ab circuits and upper body workouts, but switch to cycling, rowing or skiing machines for the warm-up and cool-down (as long as they are comfortable; movements that involve straight line movement and no impact are fine). If comfortable use these activities for the cardio workout too.

2 After a week go back to the program, including running and lower body workout. Make sure to follow good technique, particularly with lunges and squats. If your knee is fine – you are fine! Just make sure not to increase the exercise too quickly in the future.

3 If you continue to experience pain, book an appointment with a sports physio. Minor injuries indicate 'maltracking' between the joints of the knees, and if you don't do anything to correct this, the cumulative effect over the years could be osteoarthritis – a chronic degeneration of joint cartilage and the adjacent bone that can cause pain and stiffness and is a major cause of disability in later years. With the right advice, bad biomechanics can often be corrected easily – such as with a wedge of foam under the outside of the foot, or arch supports in your trainers.

4 Don't even think of wearing a knee bandage. They just push the kneecap harder against the thigh bone so every time you bend and straighten your knee the pressure of bone on bone is worse, and this will wear away the protective fluid between the knee joint. Knee bandages should only be worn under physio's advice.

5 Check your trainers. Buying a different pair may help correct maltracking (see Chapter 5, 'Do Your Prep – Get Your Kit Together'.)

stabilizing the knee

If your knee is prone to problems, stop them before they start with strengthening exercises:

1. Sit on the edge of a table with both legs dangling beneath you. Stretch out one leg until horizontal with the floor, hold this position for a few seconds, then lower. Aim for 3 sets of 10 reps, alternating legs after each lift.
2. Lie on your front with head on your hands and lift left foot to left buttock, keeping the thigh on the floor. Do 3 sets of 10 reps, alternating legs after each left. Keep your abdominals pulled in and the pelvis is static as you lift and lower, so that you isolate the hamstring.
3. These first two exercises will together strengthen the muscles that support the kneecap, building much-needed protection around the joint.
4. Work on core stability (see Chapter 7, 'The Workouts') which helps prevent knee problems – when your hips are well controlled, your pelvis doesn't go out of alignment as you move and your knee is protected. Yoga, Pilates and Core stability classes can all help.

the injury – acute knee pain

The knee is held together by four strong ligaments, all of which can be prone to injury. Ligament injuries tend to occur in sports involving dynamic sideways movements, such as rugby and skiing.

The most common injury is a sprained medial collateral ligament (MCL), where the knee moves too far towards the inside of the body. Straining the lateral collateral ligament (LCL) is much less common. Both problems are less likely if you pay attention to correct form with lower body exercises such as sumo squats, box steps and lunges. Make sure to position your knee joint in the correct way and do the movements in a slow and controlled fashion to protect the knee and avoid injury.

Also be aware of your own personal range of movement. You may not be able to squat or lunge as deeply as the diagrams indicate at first, but flexibility and strength will develop in the knee joint over time, so listen to your body and be patient.

The most severe injury is stretching your anterior cruciate ligament (ACL), an agonizing injury. There is very little chance of you suffering from an ACL injury on this program – it is rapid deceleration, seen when skis hit rocks, or in sports such as volleyball and basketball, that is often the cause. Around two-thirds of people with torn anterior cruciate ligaments find their knee gives way when they turn, and they usually require corrective surgery.

ACL injuries are 6 times more common in women than men as female hips increase the angle at which joints enter the knee, making them less stable (a situation which may be aggravated by weaker leg muscles, high heels and lax ligaments during ovulation).

the solution

1 The knee is a real weakling as far as sports injuries are concerned, with very little ability to repair itself effectively. See a physio as soon as possible if you suffer a traumatic injury as described above – ideally within an hour of the accident. The quicker you act, the fewer future complications you will experience.

2 While you are waiting to see a physio and pre-surgery, use ice or a TENS machine (*see* box on page 32) to help reduce pain and swelling, and limit the loss of range of motion, strength and function.

3 Do rehabilitation exercises recommended to you by your physio. It is usually possible to maintain cardiovascular fitness while you're out of action by doing straight line exercises (see 'Twisted Ankles' on page 25) and swimming (front crawl and backstroke only – no breaststroke because of the twisting movement it involves.)

4 As you recover, consider hiring an experienced personal trainer who can help you attain proper function, working alongside your physiotherapist.

how to use ice, TENS machines and heat treatments

ICE: Where ice is recommended, apply an ice pack or bag of frozen peas wrapped in a towel to the affected area for 15 minutes at a time for up to 1–2 hours over the next 2–3 days.

TENS: TENS machines are electrical stimulation devices that use pads placed over the injured area. They provide deep stimulation to muscles and nerves that help healing; these can be bought in pharmacies.

HEAT TREATMENTS: Where heat is recommended you can either wrap a hot water bottle in a towel and place over the injured area, or use a heat wrap. Heat wraps are electric heated cushions that can be bought in pharmacies. They come in different sizes – for shoulders, knees and ankles. Use as recommended – it has been found that heat (usually applied for 15 minutes at a time, and sometimes alternated with ice) aids surface healing of the muscle.

lower back pain

Nearly two-thirds of the population experience back pain at some point in their lives. Most problems are low level aches and pains caused by poor posture and weak abdominals, and can be triggered by using poor technique when lifting heavy objects or doing twisting movements in sport.

the injury – mild nagging pain

Mild nagging back pain ranges from general strain (which you may feel when sitting in the same position for long periods) to pulled muscles. In some instances you may also experience sharp pain radiating down the leg in a narrow band.

the solution

1 Release the pressure on your back by doing a few minutes of the back stretch (*see* point 4 below) morning and evening, followed by 10 repetitions of the back strengthening exercise in the ab circuit. A Finnish study found men who lacked strength in the lower back were 3–4 times as likely to pick up problems as those with fair or good strength.

2 Weak abs increase the odds of becoming injured because you rely more heavily on your back muscles to support you. Identify your core abdominals (*see* 'Locating Your Core', page 103) and become aware of using them in your day-to-day life, and when you are exercising. Also work on ab strength by using the ab circuit.

3 If you suspect your problems are the result of poor posture, then consider going to yoga, Pilates or Alexander technique classes that will help teach you good posture, and correct any muscle imbalances.

4 Keep your spine active during the day, by getting up from your desk every 20–30 minutes and altering your position regularly. Try this spine stretch while seated at your desk: lock your fingers together and push your arms out in front of you at chest level, drop head down with your chin on chest and pull your abs in. Hold for 10 seconds then relax.

5 If experiencing severe pain, avoid the impact sections of this program such as plyometrics, the Challenge and running.

6 If none of the above help, or if the pain worsens or brings about associated problems such as pain running down the outside of the thigh, see a physiotherapist or osteopath for a postural assessment, diagnosis and rehabilitative treatment.

the injury – acute back pain

Acute pain is likely to be due to a torn disc, impinged nerve or locked joint. Pain will be severe – something you have never felt before, like a knife in your back.

the solution

1 Contact a physiotherapist or osteopath immediately. Acute back injuries will not go into spontaneous remission and they need treatment.

2 While waiting for an appointment, try to bring down swelling and inflammation with the use of TENS and contrast (hot and cold) baths (*see* 'Stiff and Sore', page 38). When sitting choose a firm chair that encourages correct posture and helps minimize discomfort.

3 Follow the rehabilitation program given to you to the letter – if you try and speed up recovery from injuries such as a ruptured disc, you'll risk ruining the entire recovery process. Don't panic – you'll be able to regain your fitness and strength when you're fully recovered.

shin pain

the injury

Shin pain is often referred to as 'shin splints' which is a bit of a misnomer – stress fractures in the bone are rare, and it's much more likely shin pain is due to inflammation in the muscles on the shin. It is generally caused by too much running on hard surfaces or by high intensity plyometrics. It is unlikely you will experience this doing the volume of work on this program, but advice is given here just in case.

the solution

1 Apply ice to the shin if there is any visible inflammation (there may not be). Apply for 15 minutes at a time for up to 1–2 hours a day over the next 2–3 days.

2 Use a TENS machine or heat pad to aid healing.

3 Rest from impact activities for a few days – avoid running and jumping.

4 When you go back to impact activities, run on shock-absorbent surfaces (such as grass or a treadmill).

5 If the problem recurs, consider buying new trainers (from a specialist shop), or seeing a physio who can provide treatment and supply orthotics that will correct any biomechanical abnormalities.

shoulder pain

Shoulder injuries are common – the shoulder is a very unstable joint. It also has the greatest range of movement of all the body's joints, increasing its susceptibility to injury. Women have naturally looser shoulder joints than men, and the extra flexibility can make them more prone to problems.

the injury

Shoulder injuries generally involve torn or sprained muscles in the rotator cuff, a group of supporting muscles. Bad technique, muscle imbalance and lifting too heavy weights are common causes of problems.

Some shoulder injuries will recover with the care advised below, but if you suspect an acute problem – symptoms include severe pain, pain at night and pain that radiates into the neck or upper arm – you may want to see a physiotherapist.

the solution

1 Apply ice to the swelling for 15 minutes, and then apply heat for another 15 minutes. Alternate a few times and continue this treatment for 2–3 days.
2 Note your symptoms, and what positions of the arm aggravate or relieve pain. Write this down, so that if you do have to see a physiotherapist you will be able to give them as much information as possible.
3 Continue with the program but don't do anything that hurts – keep movements within pain-free ranges.
4 See a physio if things do not improve.

pulled muscles

When you pull a muscle it is usually the result of asking your body to do something that it is not used to doing. Pulled muscles can result from any high intensity physical training, including this program. Follow this program as it is set up and injuries are less likely to happen – the program has been designed with injury prevention in mind to give your body time to adapt to the changes in intensity and difficulty.

How long you'll be out of action depends on what muscle you've pulled. Groin strain (which is more likely from avoiding a tackle in rugby than doing anything on this program) takes the longest to recover, because the area gets least circulation, and can put you out of action for 6 weeks. Calf strain (from hiking uphill) tends to heal quite quickly – about 3 weeks.

Warming up can significantly reduce your chance of pulling a muscle, because oxygen consumption increases the blood supply to muscles, making them more elastic and better able to handle the stop–start and directional change movements that cause problems. Dehydration also makes muscles vulnerable to pulling, so make sure you are drinking enough water.

the injury

Pulled muscles occur when a muscle is overloaded and then ruptures, tears and bleeds internally. They are more common when muscles go into explosive muscle activity 'cold' – when the force on it exceeds its elastic capacity, it snaps much like an elastic band. If you pull a muscle then you'll normally experience a sharp soreness that makes you not want to do particular movements.

the solution

1 Apply ice to the muscle for 15 minutes, then apply heat for 15 minutes. Do a couple of cycles of this, once or twice a day for 3–4 days. This will help reduce swelling and bruising and speed up recovery.
2 Rest the affected limb for 2–3 days, and reintroduce movements as comfortable. Be gentle – don't force your body to do things that hurt.
3 If pain or symptoms worsen you should see a physiotherapist as the problem may be worse than just a strain or pulled muscle.

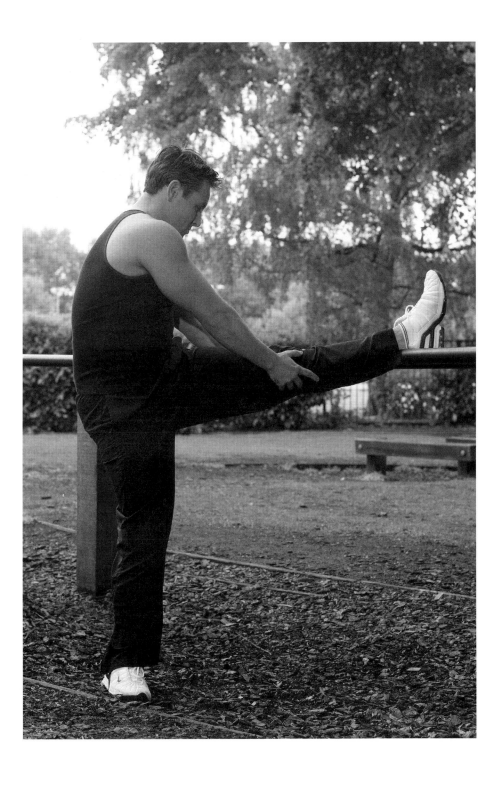

stiff and sore

the injury

Lactic acid is a by-product of exercise. Over time bodies adapt and tolerate lactic acid build-up, but when you start out on a new exercise program you may experience soreness. The programs in this book will condition the body in such a way that it adapts to muscle soreness, but you can expect it when you start.

You'll also feel stiff and sore for another reason. During training muscle tissue is broken down, causing lots of micro-tears. In rest periods fibres repair and grow, ultimately stronger. But they can feel a bit battered about in the process.

the solution

1 Use contrast baths to ease stiffness. Intersperse short periods (15–30 minutes) of the injury in warm water (not boiling hot) with periods of cold water (not freezing cold), then back into warm 2–3 times per day. Alternating hot and cold promotes healing.
2 Nutrition is important while muscles repair and grow and you need to make sure you are taking in enough of the right type of nutrients (*see* Chapter 4, 'The Body Challenge Eating Plan').
3 Carry on with your workouts when you are stiff but don't use the very sore muscles so intensely. Gentle exercise that gets blood to the affected area will help ease stiffness. So if your lower body is very stiff, train the upper body or abs the next day, using the warm-up to gently exercise the legs. In general, it's possible to train when you're stiff, but listen to your body – if you're extremely sore leave it for another day.

key points

■ Don't overtrain.

■ Increase workload gradually.

■ Be preventative – warm up, cool down, stretch and take rest days.

■ Pay attention to pain. Listen to your body and find out what it is trying to tell you.

■ Always maintain a positive outlook.

the body challenge eating plan

What you eat and drink is vital to your success during the Body

Challenge. Whether you wish to gain muscle, lose fat or get fit,

you need a diet that meets the tough demands of your training

program, and keeps your body in peak condition. Get the

nutritional balance right and you'll have plenty of energy to

power you through intense workouts. If you want to keep up

with the pace, you need to eat smart and work hard.

What you eat the day before, during and after your workout dictates how much energy you will have for your next workout and how well you will perform. Rather like filling your car up with petrol before a journey, you need to ensure your muscles are well fuelled before working out. Eat the right balance of carbohydrates, protein and healthy fats and you'll be able to keep going longer, harder and recover faster. Get it wrong and you'll soon find yourself slowing down and quickly reaching fatigue.

Getting and staying lean is a key goal of your Body Challenge. And, let's face it; a well-toned physique with good muscle definition never harmed anyone's confidence! Clearly diet plays a big part when it comes to shedding those surplus pounds. But don't become obsessed with dieting or embark on faddy weight-loss diets.

The most common mistake I see my clients make when trying to lose weight is cutting their food intake too drastically and ending up eating way too few calories. If you half-starve yourself, you won't have enough energy to get through a workout, your metabolism will slow down, you'll feel tired all the time and you'll burn hard-earned muscle. You still have to fuel your body properly even if you want to lose weight. The easiest way to lose fat and keep it off is regular intense exercise plus a healthy and careful calorie intake. Here's how to do it.

the building blocks of good sports nutrition

The more you know about food, the easier it is to make wise choices. This chapter contains a blueprint for how to eat on this program, but to make good food choices you need to know a bit more about your body's nutritional needs.

carbohydrates for energy

Carbohydrates are your main source of energy. On the Body Challenge Eating Plan, aim to get most of your carbohydrates from unprocessed fibre-rich foods that provide a slow energy release – fruit, vegetables, whole grains, beans, potatoes, brown rice and sweet corn. In this form, carbs come with a package of other nutrients, vitamins, minerals and fibre.

For main meals it is recommended you eat a portion of carbohydrate the size of your fist, combined with protein and some healthy fat (such as rice and beans). For snacks it's also good to combine carbs with protein (for instance, have an apple with a handful of nuts or a yoghurt-based smoothie) to ensure you'll get a nice steady energy release.

Go easy on 'fast carbs'. Processed sugary or starchy carbs such as biscuits, cakes, confectionery, white bread, sweetened breakfast cereals and muesli bars have a high glycaemic index, which means they produce a rapid surge of glucose in your bloodstream. This energy buzz is usually only short-lived as your pancreas pumps out insulin to bring your blood sugar levels back down. Sometimes, it over-compensates and your blood sugar levels dip too low, resulting in fatigue and hunger.

protein for muscle growth

Protein helps muscle growth and people who work out need more protein than inactive people. Skimping on protein can cause fatigue and slow recovery after workouts.

You can't build a building without adequate raw materials. It's pretty much the same when it comes to building a lean strong body – without enough protein, you won't be able to build muscle. Include a fist-sized portion of lean protein with each main meal – chicken, fish, lean meat, eggs, cottage cheese, tofu, quorn, beans, lentils or nuts.

There are 9 essential amino acids in protein foods that help muscle growth. These are all in animal proteins, soya and quorn. But plant proteins (pulses, cereals, nuts) contain smaller amounts so they need to be combined together (eg, beans on toast; lentils and rice, peanut butter on bread) to make a full complement of amino acids. The general rule of thumb is to have grains and pulses or nuts and grains together.

healthy fats for healthy tissues

Very low fat diets are a thing of the past. Not only are they bad for your health but also they won't necessarily make you lose weight! A moderate intake of healthy fat is better for you and is associated with better long-term weight control.

However, you must eat the right kind of fat. It is the heart-healthy *monounsaturated fats* (olive oil, nuts, seeds, avocados and rape seed oil) and *essential omega-3 fats* (oily fish, walnuts, omega-3-rich oils and omega-3 eggs) that can help you train smarter and get leaner. They increase the delivery of oxygen to exercising muscles, optimizing your aerobic capacity, increasing your endurance and, ultimately, helping burn more body fat. Aim to eat 1–2 portions oily fish (sardines, mackerel, salmon) a week or 1 tablespoon of an omega-3-rich oil (walnut, flax seed, rape seed, pumpkin seed) daily. If you don't eat fish, try omega-3 eggs (produced by hens fed a natural omega-3-rich seed diet) and increase intake of nuts and seeds.

At the same time as eating healthy fats, cut down on *saturated (animal) fats* (fatty meat, full-fat dairy products, butter and any products made with palm oil or palm kernel oil) and *processed (hydrogenated) fats* (margarine, low fat spreads, pastries, pies, biscuits, cereal bars, breakfast bars, cakes and bakery products, ice cream, desserts and puddings). Studies show that re-balancing your fat intake in this way not only helps weight loss but also can improve oxygen delivery to your cells, boost your metabolism and lower your blood cholesterol.

fruit and vegetables for all-round energy and health

Eat your greens … and reds, purples, yellows and oranges. Everyone should try to eat at least 5 different coloured fruit and vegetables every day. Each colour relates to different plant nutrients, each having a different health benefit. The more intense the colour, the greater the antioxidant content. These work with vitamins and minerals in the fruit and vegetables to protect your body from degenerative diseases (such as heart disease and cancer), boost immunity and fight harmful bacteria and viruses.

- **Orange/yellow foods** – carrots, apricots and mangoes contain beta-carotene;

- **Red foods** – tomatoes and watermelon are rich in lycopene, which protects against several cancers;

- **Green foods** – broccoli, cabbage and spinach are rich in magnesium, iron and chlorophyll – a terrific antioxidant;

- **Red/purple foods** – plums, cherries, red grapes, blackberries and strawberries get their colour from anthocyanins, which are even more powerful than vitamin C at fighting harmful free radicals;

- **White foods** – apples, pears and cauliflower contain flavonols, which protect against heart disease and cancer.

6 things that can sabotage your eating plan

skipping meals

Never skip meals no matter how busy you are. Leaving gaps longer than 4 hours between meals not only saps your energy but can also result in muscle loss as your body turns to protein for fuel. The Body Challenge Eating Plan is based on breakfast, lunch and evening meals, with 2 or 3 healthy snacks in between.

evening gorging

Forget big evening meals if you want to get and stay lean! Most of the calories will be stored as body fat. Many people skip breakfast and grab a sandwich at lunch, and consume most of their daily calories with a big meal in the evening. On this program aim to eat the majority of your daily calories during the morning and afternoon – spread over breakfast, lunch and 2 or 3 snacks – and eat little in the evening. This will up your metabolic rate and promote fat burning.

not drinking enough

You can easily become dehydrated over successive days of training if you fail to rehydrate fully between workouts. Symptoms of mild dehydration include fatigue, headache, loss of appetite, light-headedness and nausea – as well as lower energy levels and less endurance during training. You need to drink 1½–2 litres daily plus extra during and after your workouts (*see* 'Think Drink', page 50).

eating quick-fix foods

Fast foods, processed snacks and soft drinks are chock-a-block full of sugar, saturated fat and salt – all great energy sappers. They don't fill you up or satisfy your appetite so it's all too easy to consume too many calories. Instead, plan your diet around nutritious low glycaemic index (GI) foods that are rich in vitamins, minerals and fibre, and produce stable blood sugar levels (*see* opposite).

drinking too much alcohol

Alcohol can encourage fat storage. It is high in calories, puts undue stress on the liver and can hinder your recovery after intense workouts. Stick to safe intakes – less than 21 weekly units for men and 14 for women (1 unit is half a pint of ordinary beer or a small glass of wine).

caffeine

Drinking too much coffee, tea and other caffeinated drinks throughout the day can sap your energy and leave you feeling irritable, restless and with a headache. This is because caffeine is a stimulant that mimics the effects of stress on your body. Aim to cut down to no more than 3 cups of coffee daily. If you normally drink more, cut back gradually, otherwise you may get withdrawal symptoms such as persistent headaches.

glycaemic index – keeping your blood sugar balanced and your energy levels high

The key to keeping up your energy levels throughout your workout, as well as during the rest of the day, is to balance your blood sugar levels. Remember:

- Choose foods that have a low Glycaemic Index and give a slow blood sugar boost, such as oats, beans, lentils, vegetables and fruit. Slow burn foods and meals help improve appetite regulation and increase feelings of fullness.
- Cut down on those fast-releasing high GI carbs that cause rapid rises in blood sugar – white bread, soft drinks and sugary cereals.
- Avoid eating high GI foods on their own. Combine carbs such as bread, potatoes and white rice with protein or healthy fats to lower the overall glycaemic effect and produce a more sustained energy release. For example, have potatoes with tuna or a drizzle of olive oil rather than potatoes on their own.

The effect various foods have on blood glucose levels is measured by their glycaemic index (GI). This is a ranking of food from 0–100 that tells you how that food will affect your blood glucose levels. Glucose has the top score of 100, which means that it produces the biggest rise in blood glucose. High GI foods produce a rapid rise in blood glucose. Foods that break down more slowly, releasing glucose gradually into the bloodstream, have a low GI. The GI of various foods is given below.

High GI = 60–100
Medium GI = 40–59
Low GI = less than 40

Food	GI	Food	GI
Breakfast Cereals		*Fruit*	
Cornflakes	84	Raisins	64
Rice Crispies	82	Banana	55
Weetabix	69	Kiwi fruit	52
Muesli	56	Grapes	46
Porridge	42	Orange	44
		Apples	38
Cereal foods		Pear	38
Rice – white	87	Apricot (dried)	31
Rice – brown	76		
Pasta	45	*Snacks*	
		Crisps	54
Bread, cake and biscuits		Peanuts	14
Rice cakes	85		
White bread	70	*Dairy products*	
Wholemeal bread	69	Ice cream	61
Pizza	60	Milk – whole	27
Digestive biscuits	59	Yoghurt, fruit (low fat)	33
Sponge cake	46	Milk – skimmed	32
Vegetables		*Confectionery*	
Parsnip	97	Mars bar	68
Potato – baked	85	Muesli bar	61
Chips	75	Milk Chocolate	49
Sweet corn	55		
Carrots	49	*Drinks*	
Peas	48	Orange juice	46
		Apple juice	40
Pulses			
Baked beans	48		
Red kidney beans	27		
Lentils	26		

eating to reduce post-exercise soreness and to speed recovery

Now you're in hard training, your need for protein, omega-3 fats, B vitamins, vitamin C, beta-carotene, vitamin E, calcium, iron and zinc will be increased. Choose nutrient-rich foods – as a guide, the fresher and closer a food is to its natural state (the less it has been processed), the richer in nutrients it will be. Steaming rather than boiling food will preserve nutrients.

Make sure you're getting enough omega-3 fats, which help speed recovery after hard training and reduce inflammation and joint stiffness (*see* 'Healthy Fats for Healthy Tissues' on page 44). And try taking an antioxidant supplement (*see* 'Antioxidants' on page 53) to speed your recovery. If you suffer from stiff or painful joints, glucosamine and chondroitin supplements may help keep your joints lubricated.

before, during and after your workout

What and when you eat in relation to your workout makes a big difference to your energy, your performance and how much body fat you burn.

Eat a snack or light meal 2–4 hours before working out to give you energy for your workout, to prevent hunger, help you workout harder, prevent the shakes and stop you breaking down muscle tissue as a food source. You should feel comfortable – not full and not hungry. Suggested meals on this program all give slow-burning energy, or you can try one of the pre-workout snacks.

In an emergency have an apple, a few dried apricots, a handful of sultanas, a pot of yoghurt or even half a bar (25g) of chocolate 30 minutes before your workout to give you an energy boost.

Speed recovery with a carbohydrate and protein drink or snack as soon as possible after your workout, ideally within 30 minutes and no later than 2 hours. University of Texas researchers have found that eating a mixture of carbohydrate and protein speeds glycogen refuelling and boosts recovery. Eating within 2 hours is vital if you're working out on a daily basis and want to feel good tomorrow. Do it even if you are losing weight.

Try one of the suggested snacks – a couple of portions of fresh fruit with a pot of yoghurt, a meal replacement (protein–carbohydrate) shake or a sports bar (or nutrition, protein or meal replacement bar). Or make sure you have your next meal within this time frame.

Think drink. It takes about 30 minutes for the fluid to be absorbed into your bloodstream, so on this program what you drink before you work out will have more effect on your performance than what you drink during it. *Don't wait until you feel thirsty as this indicates that you are already on your way to dehydration! The more you sweat the more you need to drink.* The American Dietetic Association and American College of Sports Medicine recommend 150–350ml every 15–20 minutes of exercise. Choose water for workouts lasting less than 1 hour; diluted fruit juice (50/50) or an isotonic sports drink after longer workouts. Afterwards, drink little and often until your urine is pale yellow.

meal replacement bars and protein shakes

If you struggle fitting regular meals into your schedule and often have to eat on the move you can use meal replacement shakes and bars. Try to select products that are nutritious and well balanced and avoid those containing large amounts of refined sugar or fat. As a guide, choose whey-based protein shakes with multidextrin carbohydrates and a mix of vitamins and minerals. Don't worry too much about the extra little bits like amino acids – they won't make too much difference to your performance. Also, be aware that a yoghurt/milk fruit smoothie is equivalent to a protein shake, and is just as healthy.

meal plans

The key to success on this program is to plan ahead and shop for your meals in advance. Don't rely on getting the right foods from restaurants, takeaways or even the gym. Each day, you should have 3 meals (breakfast, lunch and an evening meal) and 2–3 healthy snacks. Here are some meal suggestions.

breakfasts

- Wholemeal toast with honey or peanut butter and a carton of yoghurt;
- Porridge made with skimmed milk, topped with raisins and pumpkin seeds (try flaxseeds and sunflower seeds too);
- Cereals such as Muesli, Weetabix or Shredded wheat with skimmed milk and fresh fruit;
- Fresh fruit salad with natural yoghurt and sunflower seeds;
- Toasted bagel with low-fat cream cheese and fresh fruit;
- Boiled or poached egg with wholemeal toast.

mid-morning snack

- Fresh fruit;
- Homemade or ready-bought smoothie;
- Handful of almonds, cashews, walnuts or seeds;
- Meal replacement shake;
- Handful of trail mix.

lunch

- Pasta with tomato sauce, sprinkle of grated cheese and side salad;
- Wholemeal sandwich with chicken, prawns or egg and salad;
- Jacket potato with chilli beans, tuna or cottage cheese and salad;
- Grilled fish, chicken or cooked beans with rice and steamed vegetables;
- Chicken, bean or lentil soup with wholemeal roll and fruit;
- Wholemeal roll, pitta bread or wrap filled with turkey and salad;
- Pasta with tuna and sweet corn;
- Baked beans on toast and salad;

- Hummus with pitta bread, vegetable crudités and avocado slices;
- Smoked salmon with salad.

mid-afternoon snack

- Sports (meal replacement or protein) bar or breakfast bar;
- Rice cakes with peanut butter;
- Fresh fruit with yoghurt;
- Milkshake made with skimmed milk, fresh fruit and yoghurt;
- Mixed sunflower and sesame seeds and raisins.

evening meal

- Grilled or baked fish (salmon, mackerel or trout) with jacket potato (optional) and steamed vegetables;
- Prawn or marinated tofu and vegetable stir-fry with wholegrain rice (optional);
- Grilled chicken or turkey breast with salad and new potatoes (optional);
- Turkey, lentil or quorn and vegetable curry;
- Chicken or vegetable paella;
- Mixed bean chilli with salad;
- Lentil and vegetable soup;
- Bolognese made with turkey or beef mince or quorn with pasta and vegetables;
- Kebabs made with lean meat or marinated tofu, peppers, courgettes, mushrooms and tomatoes, and wholegrain rice (optional);
- Grilled sardines (or other oily fish) with grilled Mediterranean vegetables.

supplements

Remember supplements should not replace a healthy diet. Take them in addition to – not instead of – normal eating and they may help to give you the edge.

antioxidants

Antioxidant supplements contain various combinations of beta-carotene, vitamin C, vitamin E, selenium, zinc, magnesium, lycopene (the red pigment found in tomatoes) and anthocyanidins (plant pigments). They help boost your body's defences to fight potentially harmful free radicals and protect against heart disease, cancer and the ageing process. They may also promote recovery after intense workouts and reduce post-exercise soreness.

creatine

Creatine is a protein that combines with phosphorus to form phosphor-creatine in your muscles, a high-energy compound that fuels intense exercise. Supplements may help increase strength, muscle mass and performance and are popular with those doing high-intensity workouts such as sprinters and weightlifters, but be warned, studies show that they don't work for everyone. Try taking daily doses of 3–6g for 30 days, divided into 4 equal doses, at mealtimes. The accompanying carbohydrates helps drive creatine into the muscles.

glucosamine

If you suffer from joint problems, glucosamine may help alleviate stiffness and joint pain. It is a cartilage-building sugar compound that's made naturally in the body. Supplements help prevent the progression of cartilage damage and stimulate cartilage repair. The recommended dose is 500 mg, 3 times a day. Choose a supplement that combines glucosamine with omega-3 fish oil as this also promotes healthy joints.

glutamine

Taking glutamine immediately after intense workouts may help you recover faster, reduce muscle soreness and cut your risk of catching colds and other infections.

multivitamins and minerals

During hard training, your requirements for many vitamins and minerals will be higher than the recommended daily allowances (RDAs) for the general population so supplements may help you meet your needs better. But remember, supplements do not make up for a poor diet.

essential oil supplements

Taking a daily supplement rich in omega-3 oils is a good way of boosting your daily intake, especially as there are only a few foods that are naturally rich in these oils. To boost your energy levels, improve performance and speed fat loss, include a tablespoon of an omega-3-rich oil (such as walnut or flax seed oil) or a blend based on flax seed oil, and use in salad dressings or stirred into soups and sauces. Alternatively, take up to 8 capsules of omega-3 or marine fish oil daily.

serious strength – 5 eating tips for building muscle

1 **Get your calories right**. Building serious muscle requires extra fuel so you'll need to increase the size of your portions. Add an extra 500 calories to your usual daily diet if you're a hard gainer.
2 **Step up protein**. You'll need more protein, too. Aim for 1.4–1.8g protein for each kg of your body weight – that's about 98–126g if you weigh 70kg. Increase protein portions by about one fifth.
3 **Eat 6 meals a day**. Get into the habit of eating every 2–3 hours, that's 3 meals and at least 2–3 healthy snacks. This will provide a near-constant influx of protein, carbohydrates and other nutrients to build muscle.
4 **Try a supplement**. Meal replacement and protein shakes on top of your normal eating are a good way of boosting your nutritional intake. Most contain whey protein – derived from milk – which may also boost your immune system and protect against muscle breakdown during intense training.
5 **Fuel your body with protein and carbs 1 hour after working out**. Researchers have found that protein combined with carbohydrate promotes

faster glycogen refuelling and greater muscle mass gains. Good post-workout snacks include a tuna sandwich, a meal replacement shake or bar, yoghurt or a jacket potato with cottage cheese.

fat burners – 5 tips for fat loss

1 **Practice portion control**. Cut back your portion sizes by about 15%. As a rule of thumb, the carbohydrate and protein portions should be no bigger than the size of your fist.

2 **Cut back carbs in the evening**. Reducing starchy foods after 5 pm is a good way of keeping your calorie intake down. Go easy on potatoes, bread and pasta. Try to eat a smaller meal comprised mainly of healthy vegetables and lean protein. Avoid eating altogether 2 hours before you go to bed.

3 **Time your meals for greater fat burning**. The general rule on this program is to eat 2–4 hours before you work out, or snack 30 minutes before in emergencies. If you're a fat burner, avoid eating anything within 2–3 hours beforehand. This will force your body to dip into its fat stores. (But don't forget to eat altogether – otherwise you'll just flake out!)

4 **Wait 1 hour after your workout before eating**. The general rule on this program is to eat within 2 hours of working out. Fat burners should wait 1 hour before consuming anything, because during this time the body will continue to burn fat to replenish fuel reserves.

5 **Have a good breakfast**. Eating a good carbohydrate-based breakfast, with some protein, to kick-start your metabolism in the morning. Those carbs will be used to fuel your daily activities and workouts instead of being stored as fat. Skipping breakfast increases the chances of snacking on high-calorie foods later in the day.

easy calorie swaps

Replace	With	Calories saved
1 oz cheese	½ oz very strong cheese	70–10
Oil for cooking	Oil spray	120 per tbsp
Pain au chocolate	2 slices wholemeal toast with Marmite or similar spread	100
Buttered/sweet popcorn	Salted popcorn	95 per 75g portion
Crisps	Twiglets or similar low-fat snacks	50 per 25g bag
2 chocolate biscuits	2 rice cakes with jam	60
Shop-bought meat lasagne	Vegetable lasagne	173 per 420g portion
Chicken korma	Chicken tikka	230 per 350g portion
Chocolate bar	Breakfast or cereal bar	150
Cola	Water	136 per 330ml can
Creamy fruit yoghurt	Very low fat yoghurt	119 per 150g pot
1 pint of lager	1 glass dry white wine	74
1 glass fruit juice	1 glass half juice/half water	50

key points

- Food is fuel. Give your body the best and you'll achieve the best results.

- Eat 3 main meals a day, each containing protein to build muscle and carbo-hydrate to provide you with plenty of energy.

- Eat 2 healthy snacks a day in-between your main meals. These will keep your energy levels up.

- Drink at least 2 litres of water a day.

- Plan and shop for your meals in advance – don't rely on getting the right foods from a restaurant or takeaway.

- Choose fresh nutrient-dense unprocessed foods to give your body vitamins, minerals and fibre.

- Learn the difference between good fats and bad fats, and make sure you're getting enough omega-3 fats, which help speed recovery.

- Maximize training results and energy for the next day by having a carbo-hydrate and protein drink or snack as soon as possible after your workout. Ideally within 30 minutes, and no later than 2 hours.

do your prep – get your kit together

Preparation is important before you start this regime – you don't want workouts to be time consuming. The whole philosophy of this program is about being able to warm up, workout, cool down and stretch in just over 30 minutes, so spending 10 minutes finding your kit, locating your trainers, feeding the dog and answering the phone – it's not on! You'll work out more if you don't spend time dithering around wondering where your things are.

In the previous chapters you've learnt how to switch off from work and switch on to your workout, and to plan (and prepare) meals in advance. So there's just one final thing – making sure you have the right trainers and kit there at the end of your bed when you wake up in the morning.

always prepare the night before

If your kit is prepared and laid out then you'll get out there, even if you're still sleepy. But the more you have to think about it, the more likely it is you'll decide you don't have time … *Preparation eliminates thinking time.*

equipment needed

trainers

One pair of good running trainers are all you need for this program. There's an argument for buying two – then you can alternate them from day to day, which is supposed to increase their longevity – but it's not essential.

When you run your feet experience the impact of 3–7 times your body weight, so finding a shoe that provides motion control and cushioning can lessen the stress on your joints. Don't try to become an expert in biomechanics yourself, go to a specialist running shop where they will have a look at your running style – outside, or on a treadmill in the shop – and guide you through a custom fitting process to help you stay injury free.

The most important element about one's feet is how they pronate – that is, how the arch side of your foot rolls inward and drops down when you run. This is one of the key ways your body absorbs shock. Approximately 70% of runners pronate properly, 25% of runners pronate excessively, while 5% do not pronate enough.

Those who pronate enough are classified as having neutral biomechanics and require neutral (sometimes called stability) running shoes. These allow the foot to follow its normal motion.

People who pronate excessively are classified as overpronators and require motion-control shoes that support the arch and reduce the motion of your feet. (Without this, overpronators can experience heel pain, shin pain, knee pain, Achilles tendonitis, hip and low back pain).

Finally, there are those who do not pronate enough and they are called supinators or underpronators. Remember, pronation means shock absorption and since supinators don't pronate enough, they don't absorb shock properly and therefore need a cushioned shoe. Supinators are prone to stress-related injuries including anterior shin pain (outside of the shin).

Once you have worked out a style of shoe to fit your biomechanics, try on a few models to find a proper fit. Key things to look for are a wide enough forefront and snug heel.

kit

It's not up to me to tell you what to wear, but whatever your style statement, observe a few rules:

1 Wear things that are comfortable and allow your body to breathe. Your outfit should not be a distraction.
2 Do not buy clothes that are restrictive. Choose stretchy fabrics in suitable sizes.
3 Buy proper sports clothing so you feel properly sporty – wearing a baggy grey T-shirt and saggy tracksuit pants will make you feel tired, fat and useless.
4 Buy proper socks that allow your feet to breathe, don't cramp the toes, and are blister preventative – 1000-miles socks, for example, provide good cushioning.

water bottle

The more hydrated you are the more energetic you'll feel, and refuelling with water during your workout can help keep energy up. Buy a bottle that allows you to slide your hand through it to carry on runs, or a waist pouch to put it in.

barbell or dumbbells

All you need is a set of dumbbells to do this workout at home. Choose a set of different weights, and choose metal over plastic as they last longer.

If you want to invest in a barbell set too, choose ones with a slide lock (*not* a screw lock) so you can save time changing weights between reps.

skipping rope

You'll need a skipping rope for some of the warm-ups. Buy a plastic coated one that's easy to keep clean. Choose one with lightly-weighted handles that swings faster to maintain momentum. Skipping ropes are one size fits all – if it's too long for you shorten it by tying a knot near the handle.

optional extras

body fat monitor

Your aim on this program is to get fitter, but that doesn't necessarily mean getting lighter – muscle weighs more than fat so it's perfectly possible to revolutionize your body and still weigh the same.

This is why body fat scales are more motivating than normal scales. They work by passing small electrical currents (too weak to be sensed) through your body to measure body fat – thus helping chart the transformation of your body from fat to fit by calculating lean tissue. It's important to remember that each pound of lean muscle is firmer and more compact than a pound of fat (and burns an estimated extra 50 calories a day even when it's doing nothing).

There are a number of different fat monitors on the market and they tend to give different readings because they calculate body fat percentage using different equations. But while initial readings may vary, all are quite good at tracking changing body composition over time.

heart rate monitor

The cardio circuits in this program work on monitoring your rate of perceived exertion rather than heart rate, so you can adjust intensity easily.

However if you want to use a heart rate monitor you can. If you have high or low blood pressure then your doctor will recommend a maximum heart rate that is safe for you, and a heart rate monitor will help you keep within that limit.

sports watches

There are a number of sports watches available that will time your circuits so you don't have to – simply set the clock and it will beep every 30 seconds or minute as appropriate. Otherwise use an egg timer which buzzes every 30 seconds.

key points

- Go to a specialist running shop and get fitted out with running shoes that suit your biomechanics.

- Wear proper sports clothing and keep it clean – grubby kit won't get you fit.

- Prepare your kit the night before – preparation eliminates thinking time and makes workouts quick and efficient.

the warm-up and cool-down routines

Too busy to warm up, too macho to cool down? Big mistake!

It's essential to warm up for 5 minutes for preventing injury, and

cool-down stretches create long lean muscles with a full range of

motion. Here's how to get the whole business done effectively

and efficiently.

Time-pressed people often skip the warm-up and cool-down, thinking that because they feel easy they don't count. They do! Giving your body time to prepare and recover from exercise prevents injury and gives you fitness longevity. Warming up makes sessions easier as well as safer, and cooling down allows the heart rate to stabilize and gives the body time to repair and recover.

Since you have to spend this time warming up and cooling down, enjoy it! There's a mental edge to these sessions too. The warm-up is the part of the session where you leave all your troubles behind you and start to loosen up and look forward to the work you're about to do. The cool-down stretch is the bit where you chill out, feel the stress dissolve in some stretches and reflect on what you've achieved.

warming up

The warm-up phase is designed to increase the flow of blood and oxygen to muscles. It makes exercise feel easier; when your muscles are warm they are able to contract more easily so you can work at a higher intensity for less perceived effort.

I never let clients skip this phase because muscles become more elastic during the warm-up, reducing the chances of pulling a muscle or tearing something. Activity also pushes synovial fluid through the joints, increasing the range of movement and joint flexibility all over your body – knees, elbows, back. If you have been sedentary all day, the chances are you feel creaky; the warm-up will put life back into your body. Injuries take 3 weeks to 6 months to heal – don't put yourself at risk!

the routine

In this program the warm-up is simple: just 5 minutes of walking, slow jogging or intermittent skipping to get blood flowing through your muscles. This is sufficient to get your body ready for exercise.

People used to do stretches as a warm-up routine but fitness thinking has changed – research has found that cold muscle is easily injured. There are two exceptions to this rule:

1   If you are feeling the stresses and strains of a previous workout, add a few stretches onto the end of your warm-up to help relieve muscle pressure and make your workout more comfortable. Just make sure you are warm before you start, and stretch very gently.

2   If your shoulders or back feel tight from sitting down all day, or you know these are weak areas for you, incorporate a few light mobility exercises, such as shoulder and arm rolls, into your warm-up to help lubricate your joints and prevent injury. Going straight from static to using the treadmill, lifting heavy weights or doing dynamic movements puts a huge strain on your back and is not recommended, so lie on your back and hug your knees to your chest (*see* Lower Back stretch on page 70) until you feel comfortable.

the mindset

Use the warm-up to bring your mind and body together to work as one. As soon as you change from your work clothes to your gym clothes, that's when your focus starts. Don't even think about using preparation and recovery time to write mental shopping lists or rehash today's problems. Forget the day and its irritations, and notice how your body feels and as you relax into activity, concentrate on your ambitions for this session.

You'll get a lot more out of your workout if you decide what you want to achieve before you start. During the warm-up think about your goal, whether it's to do a certain number of reps, or to focus on doing everything with perfect form. You'll find it's a lot more rewarding exercising with awareness than doing a session with half a mind on what you're going to cook for supper and the other half on whether you want to do this session at all! You're here now, so get ready to enjoy it.

cooling down

The cool-down consists of 10 minutes of slowing down and stretching exercises to bring your heart rate gently back down to the resting heart rate, and stop you feeling faint or dizzy. The workouts all contain 5 minutes of gentle jogging, skipping or powerwalking. After this you should do the 5-minute full-body stretch (*see* page 69).

As you stretch, blood is moved into that area, helping to prevent injury and disperse the lactic acid that may have built up during the workout, helping to prevent any associated stiffness you could feel the next day.

Stretching is also important for posture and range of motion (vital to good sports performance). Every mile you run, every weight you lift, every hour you spend sitting or driving, muscles become shorter. It's called adaptive shortening, and unless you stretch they will stay short, making you feel old, ruining your posture and making everyday actions harder to perform. But just a few simple stretches can reverse this, increasing the range of motion of your muscles, helping to make life more comfortable, improve sports performance and prevent injury. This also helps create long lithe muscles that look great!

the routine

Make stretches slow, gentle and hold them for 30 seconds. You should feel a comfortable pull as you stretch. Don't bounce-stretch, or try to push or pull yourself into a deeper stretch than is comfortable – this will simply activate the stretch reflex and the muscles will contract against it, making the whole activity counterproductive. Overstretching can make muscles tired, and could injure them. Signs that you are overstretching a muscle include feeling unbearable rather than comfortable pain, and muscle shaking.

If stretching is new to you, your task for the first few weeks will be to get your muscles and connective tissues accustomed to stretching, and to enjoy the increased range of motion in crucial joints such as your hips, lower back and shoulders. As you progress, your flexibility will dramatically increase, building strength at the point where muscles are most extended – and improving performance on the squash court, climbing wall or football pitch.

You may have heard about more advanced stretching techniques, such as PNF (proprioceptive neuromuscular facilitation), but you need not concern yourself with them for this program; this simple stretch program will increase flexibility all over the body quickly and effectively.

the 5-minute full body stretch

Do these stretches after every workout, holding each for 30 seconds each. They target every muscle in the body from top to toe. All the following exercises are done standing with feet shoulder-width apart.

neck

Gently tilt the head to one side until you feel a stretch on the opposite side of the neck. Then repeat on the other side.

Tip: Increase the stretch from neck to shoulder by placing your right hand on top of your head as your head tilts to the right.

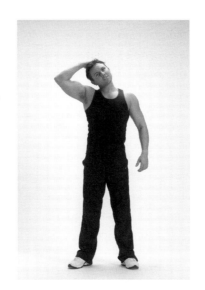

upper back

Clasp your hands together and push your arms straight out in front of you at shoulder level, parting your shoulder blades.

Tip: To create a more intense stretch, use a pole or gym machine that you can hang backwards from to increase the stretch.

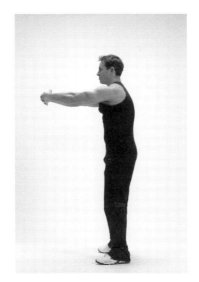

lower back

Lie on your back and pull your knees to your chest so your tailbone curves gently off the floor. Rock your knees back and forth slowly for 15 seconds. Then with hands on knees gently circle the knees clockwise, then anticlockwise for 15 seconds.

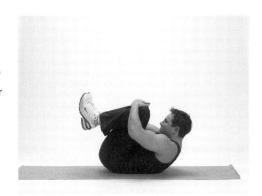

Tip: If you want to take longer doing stretches you may – you can never do too much. But the stretches I've designed here are for speed and efficiency.

chest

Hold your abdominals tight and keep your head, neck and shoulders relaxed. Clasp your hands behind your back and lift your arms behind you until you feel the stretch across your chest.

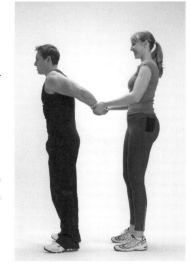

Tip: If you are working with a buddy, increase the stretch by getting them to raise your hands at the back. Don't lean forward: keep your head in the same position.

shoulders

Bend one arm and bring it across your body at shoulder height. Place your opposite hand or forearm on the upper arm and push to increase the stretch. Repeat on the other side.

Tip: Be careful not to shrug your shoulders as you do this. Keep them down and relaxed.

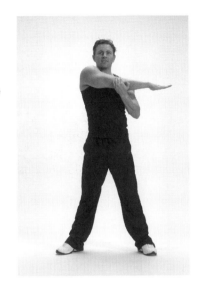

triceps

Raise your left arm in the air, bend at the elbow and place the hand behind your head in the middle of your shoulder blades. Place your right hand on the left elbow and push against your arm to increase the stretch. Keep your back and neck in alignment as you stretch. Repeat on the other side.

Tip: Push your head back on to your arm to increase the stretch slightly.

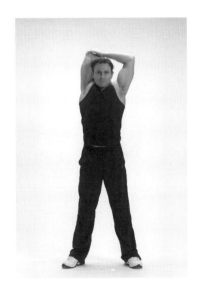

quads (front thighs) and hips

Stand up straight with one hand on a wall, chair or your workout buddy. Bend one leg at the knee, pulling your foot towards your buttock and keeping your knees together. Repeat on the other leg.

Tip: Keep your tailbone tucked under so there is a straight line down the front of your body – this will increase the stretch on your hip flexors and thighs. The supporting leg should be slightly bent.

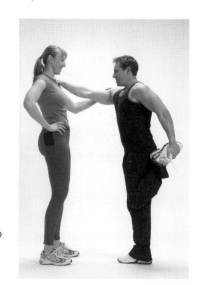

hamstring (back thighs)

Stand and place one leg straight out in front of you, with your heel on the ground and toe flexed. Bend your supporting leg slightly then bend forward from the hips, keeping your abs pulled tight. Repeat on the other leg.

Tip: To increase the stretch, bend further forward from the hips, keeping your back straight.

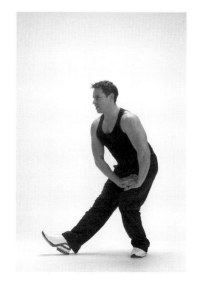

calves

Stand with your hands against the wall at shoulder height and step one foot back behind you. Keep your front leg slightly bent and the back leg straight. Push the heel of your back leg into the ground. Repeat on the other side.

Tip: Place the other foot on the back of your heel to increase the stretch.

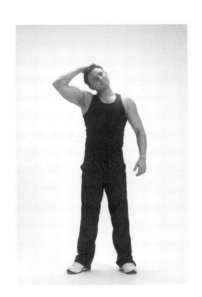

the mindset

As you stretch out, think about what you have done and congratulate yourself on it. Allow your body to feel strong. Tell yourself that you're fit, strong and flexible – even if you don't feel like it. It's mind over matter: let your mind override your body and feel the fitness high.

key points

- Always warm up, cool down and stretch. These vital parts of the workout help prevent injury, keep you flexible and give you fitness longevity.

- Get into the right frame of mind before you start. It's the key to enjoying your exercise session.

- Tell yourself that you're fit, strong and flexible. In time your body will grow towards your praise.

the workouts

Now you've prepared your kit and got psyched up for what lies ahead. The final stage of your preparation is to get to know the workouts you'll be doing over the next 4 weeks. Some of these exercises will be familiar to you already, some may be new – but in time you will be able to do them all. Follow the instructions in this chapter and soon you'll be feeling fitter and stronger than ever before.

There are 5 workouts in the program: one to strengthen and tone the lower body, one to hone and strengthen the upper body, one to sculpt abs, a cardio workout to burn fat, and a plyometrics workout that works on dynamic power. Many workout programs focus on just one of these elements of fitness, but by alternating the demands on your body by training it in three different dimensions simultaneously, you will achieve far greater results in much less time (in this case, just 30 minutes, 4 or 5 times a week).

There is a popular idea that celebs spend hours a day in the pursuit of the body beautiful. While some do, most have such busy schedules that they're looking for maximum results in minimum time. This means working hard, but not necessarily long. For her role in the Bond film *Die Another Day*, Halle Berry and I worked out for 30 minutes a day, 4 times a week. Devote the same time (and effort) and you too can have you own Bond girl (or 007) body. How long it takes depends on your starting point. Halle has great genes and had a good level of base fitness when we started, but everyone can achieve radical results in a few months on this program.

All the sessions are short, intense and effective. Whether you're a professional athlete or a professional mum, this program can be incorporated into your life and will improve your fitness.

staying focused

Trying to get fit on autopilot is like driving somewhere new when you're listening to the radio and not looking at a map – you'll probably get there eventually but it will take you a lot longer than if you focus on what you're doing! This chapter teaches you how to do the exercises properly – there's no point in going off half-cocked. The more you concentrate on good form as you work out, the greater the rewards you will see.

As a personal trainer part of my job is keeping my clients focused on form throughout their sessions. On this program it's up to you to stay mentally alert, so you know you're recruiting the right muscles for each exercise (no cheating!) and not doing anything that could cause injury. Being focused also makes workouts twice as relaxing, as you get a complete break from the rest of your life. So enjoy working out with good form, be proud of the control exercises as you lift and lower weights, and relish in the improvements you can feel in your performance as you go along.

The detailed instructions in this chapter are the ones I give to my clients. Follow them closely the first few times you do the workouts until you internalize them; then it's down to you to do your own mental checks. After a while you'll be able to use the thumbnail sketches of the workouts, but it will be worth re-reading the fuller instructions now and again to make sure you aren't getting into any bad habits. Also make use of the tips given next to each exercise; these can help you get a little bit more out of each exercise, or help you adapt the program to your existing level of fitness (for some of you, doing 10 full press-ups right now might seem as likely as climbing Everest! Don't worry – it will get easier).

functional fitness

Fitness isn't just about vanity and the body beautiful; it's about energy for life. Sure, you want to look thinner, stronger, leaner and more attractive, but you probably want to apply that body strength to your life – whether you're playing soccer, climbing mountains or running around after children.

This program uses a mixture of weights, cardio and plyometric circuits to make sure you get as functionally fit as possible. If you work out already, the chances are you do a mixture of cardio and weights already. Plyometrics, which involve explosive movements such as squat thrusts and jumps, are the circuits that will enable you to apply your new strength quickly. When you can do this you'll be able to get off the starting line quickly, accelerate up a hill, and bound over obstacles. You'll feel fit for life.

the challenge

It is strange but true that we often don't want to do tests, but afterwards we feel great that we rose to the challenge. After all, it's human nature to take on challenges – and to want to win! This is why the program includes a once-a-month plyometric circuit called 'The Challenge'. This is a 50-minute circuit that allows you to measure your increasing fitness. Just by doing it you've already passed.

lower body workout

body benefits

This workout is designed to increase strength in all the leg muscles. It will sculpt and define the shape of your legs, making them look longer and leaner, and more athletic.

The exercises are designed to work together to create balanced strength in the different muscles in the legs, to strengthen them and increase joint stability. If you've ever pulled a hamstring or had shin splints, it's probably down to muscular imbalance (with one set of leg muscles overpowering the other). These dynamic exercises train muscles together to improve balance and provide leg power, giving you the muscles you need for sculpted strong legs.

WARM-UP: 5 MINUTES

Skip or jog for 5 minutes.

the circuit

This circuit takes 4 minutes to complete. Rest for 1 minute after each circuit, then repeat. Do it 4 times, then follow with the cool-down and stretch.

While performing these exercises, remember to pull in your core abdominal muscles to protect your back and maintain good form.

SQUATS: 1 MINUTE

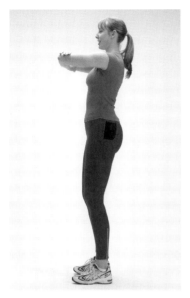

Stand with feet hip-width apart, knees slightly bent. Cross your arms and hold them out in front of you at shoulder height.

Tip: Ordinary squats take you to a 90 degree bend in your legs. For an extra challenge, lower beyond this point. This will recruit more muscles in your hamstrings and glutes – the muscles in the buttocks.

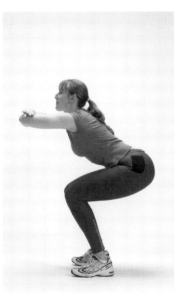

As you breathe in, lower your body as if you were sitting back on a chair, bending the knees until your thighs are parallel with the ground. Keep your abs tight, and don't let your knees move in front of your toes. Breathing out, push through your heels to return to the start position, being careful not to lock your knees. If you like, hold a barbell across the front or back of your shoulders.

ALTERNATE LUNGES: 30 SECONDS EACH LEG

Treat this as a 4-point move.

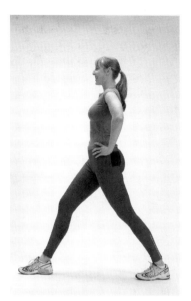

Start with both legs together, then breathe in and stride forward a good pace with your right foot.

Tip: To increase intensity, hold a dumbbell in each hand.

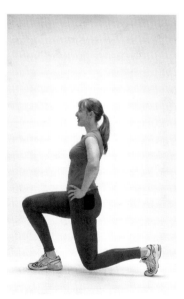

Drop down, keeping the lower half of your forward leg perpendicular to the floor, and your torso upright. Keep your tailbone curled under.

Breathe out and push up through the thigh and lower muscles of both legs. Step back to the start position, pushing through your heel, not your toes.

Repeat, stepping forward with your left leg.

SUMO SQUATS: 1 MINUTE

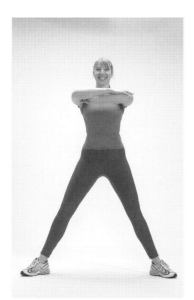

Stand with your feet just over shoulder-width apart and toes angled outwards at about 45 degrees. Cross your arms and hold them out from your body, parallel to the floor. Tuck the pelvis under, and keeping your chin tucked in and trunk erect, slowly bend your legs and squat down.

Tip: Squeeze your glutes (the muscles in your bottom) hard to increase the toning effect. Ensure you feel this in the inner thigh.

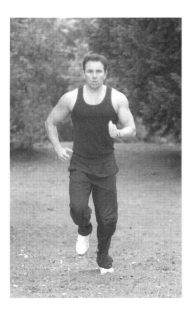

Lower yourself until your thighs are parallel to the floor. Then straighten your legs by pushing hard through the heels and repeat.

WEIGHTED STEP-UPS: 30 SECONDS EACH LEG

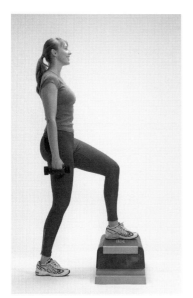

Stand facing a bench or step, with your hands by your sides holding dumbbells. Use your hands like hooks, rather than clasping the weights with your arms, so that the weight is carried as a dead weight by your legs not your upper body. Breathe out and step up with one foot, placing your whole foot on the bench.

Tip: Maintain good posture, rolling your shoulders gently back, standing tall and keeping your torso in alignment.

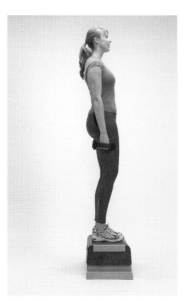

Push through your heels, and step up with your other foot so you are standing on the bench, making sure you don't lock your knees at the top. Step down with the same foot. Then repeat with the other leg.

STRAIGHT-LEG DEAD LIFT: 1 MINUTE

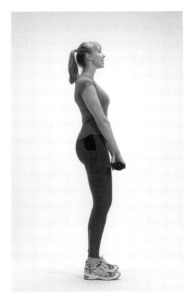

Stand up straight with your feet shoulder-width apart, holding the barbell or dumbbells with your palms facing your thighs and with your knees slightly soft. Activate your core muscles by drawing in your abdomen to protect your back.

Tip: This is the best way there is to exercise hamstrings, which carve out the curve between your thighs and buttocks. If you have a bad back you could replace this exercise with a hamstring curl machine in the gym.

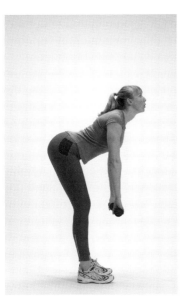

Bend forwards at the hips keeping your chest raised and head up. Lower the barbell or dumbbells to the point where you feel a slight resistance in your hamstrings. Then return to the start position, bringing you hips through at the end.

COOL-DOWN: 5 MINUTES

Walk or jog for 5 minutes. You've been using your legs intensely so if you have space, do a variety of moves to make your legs work in different directions – do the steps footballers and rugby players do along the side of the pitch: side steps, long extended steps, short springs, skips, then run kicking your heels up at the back and raising your knees at the front.

STRETCH: 5 MINUTES

Do the 5-minute full-body stretch (*see* page 69).

time taken: 35 minutes

upper body workout

body benefits

This workout trains the whole upper body, creating strong shapely muscles in the arms, back and shoulders. The upper body tends to be the weakest area, as it is used little in modern life, but it responds well to training. You'll see results in the arms and shoulders faster than in any other area of the body, and can expect visibly toned muscular arms within weeks.

These exercises provide good aesthetic returns – but they aren't just about looks. They are designed to build multipurpose muscles that work better together – this is especially important with the shoulders, which are easily injured. A strong back is essential for every great athlete – you can't throw a ball, swing a racket or climb a rock without good back muscles. This workout will stabilize the whole upper body, reducing risk of injury.

WARM-UP: 5 MINUTES

Skip or jog for 5 minutes.

the circuit

There are 8 exercises in this circuit each taking 30 seconds, so it takes 4 minutes overall. Do it once, take 1 minute's rest, then repeat. Do the whole circuit 4 times, then follow with the cool-down and stretch.

Tip: Move quickly from one exercise to the next. Make each individual movement slow and controlled – don't cheat by doing them at speed, as gravity will then be doing part of the work for you.

PRESS-UPS ON KNEES: 30 SECONDS

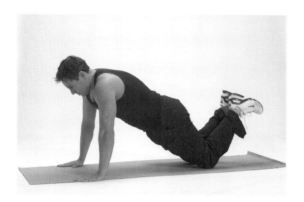

Kneel on all fours, placing your hands directly under your shoulders. Lower your hips so that there is a straight line between your knees and your shoulders. This is your starting position.

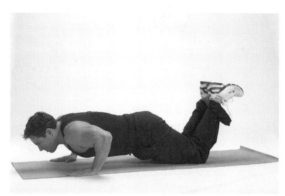

Exhale, and bend your arms and lower your body until your chest is a couple of inches off the ground (you should be able to fit an imaginary fist between your chest and the floor). Keep your back straight and don't stick your bottom in the air. Breathe in, then press back up to the start position while breathing out. Keep your abs tight throughout the movement.

Tip: The further your knees are from your hands, the harder the exercise. As soon as you are strong enough, replace these with full press-ups.

FULL PRESS-UPS: 30 SECONDS

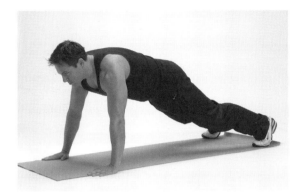

Adopt the position shown, with your knees off the floor and weight on hands and feet.

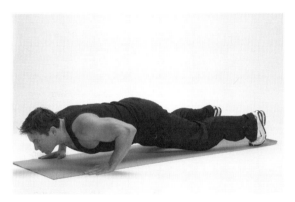

Breathe in as you bend your arms until your chest is 2 in (5 cm) off the floor, remembering to keep your back straight. Inhale, then breathe out as you return to the start position. To keep your body in strict alignment, think of a broom handle running from the top of your head through to your heels.

Tip: Vary your hand position between circuits to put the emphasis on different muscles group. Do one set with hands close together to put emphasis on the triceps, do one set with normal hands under shoulders position to put emphasis on the chest and triceps, and do one set with hands wide and fingers pointing out which puts emphasis on the shoulders. For the final set, advanced exercisers can put their hands very close together.

PULL-UPS (AIDED): 30 SECONDS

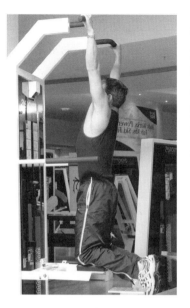

Use a pull-up machine that has a platform to support your weight. Hold the bars above your head with an overhand grip, so your hands are just wider than shoulder-width apart. Your knees should be bent and resting on the platform beneath you.

Tip: If you are doing this circuit at home, replace pull-ups with another minute of the bent-over row (*see* page 93).

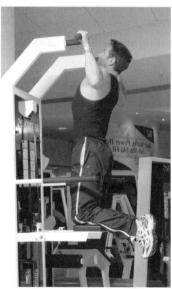

Exhale, and pull your body up until your eyes are level with the bar. Hold for 1 second, then slowly lower yourself back down to the starting position. It is important to isolate your back muscle and squeeze it at the top for optimum contraction.

TRICEP DIPS: 30 SECONDS

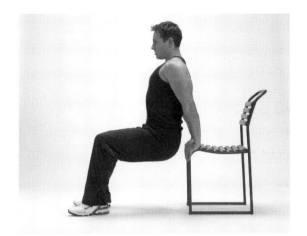

Sit on a chair or bench with your hands on the front edge of the seat, facing forward. Keeping your feet flat on the floor in front of you, slide your bottom off the bench so your weight is transferred to your arms.

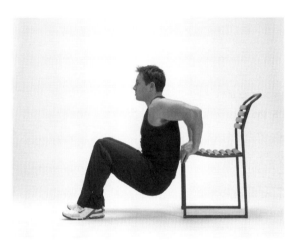

From here, inhale and lower, keeping your back close to the bench and stopping when your upper arms are parallel to the floor. Keep your elbows tucked in so they go back behind you or out to the sides. Return to the start position by straightening your arms. Do not hunch your shoulders, or lock out your elbows at the top.

Tip: Raise your legs off the floor – on a bench or another chair – to make this exercise harder.

BICEP CURLS: 30 SECONDS

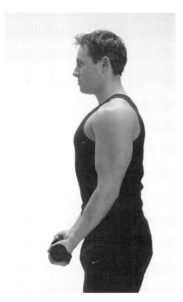

Stand with your feet hip-width apart, knees soft. Start with your arms by your sides, elbows slightly bent, holding a barbell or two dumbbells in front of you so your palms face away from your body.

Tip: If you are using a barbell, make sure you don't lean back as you lift. This is bad form and puts stress on your lower back.

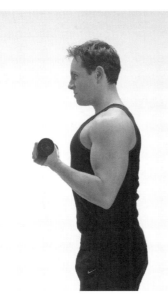

Breathe out and slowly raise the barbell (or dumbbells) to your chest, keeping your elbows tucked in close to your body. Squeeze your biceps then breathe in as you return to the start position. Raise and lower the weights at the same speed – your muscles will work harder if the movement is slow and controlled.

LATERAL RAISES: 30 SECONDS

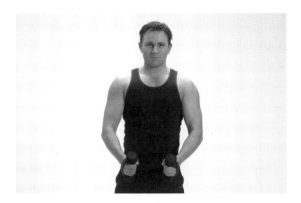

Stand with your feet hip-width apart, holding a dumbbell in each hand. Your hands should face each other.

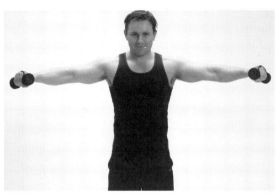

Raise the dumbbells out to the sides, at the same time turning your hands so they face the floor (as if you were pouring water from a jug). Raise them until your elbows and hands are level with your shoulders (keep your elbows bent). Slowly return to the starting position, resisting the weight on the way down.

Tip: Lead with your elbows as you raise your arms. Raise and lower your arms at the same speed.

SHOULDER PRESS: 30 SECONDS

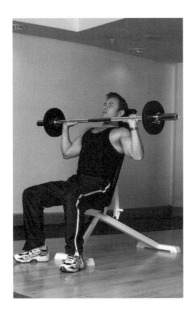

Sit on a chair or bench with your back well supported and your feet hip-width apart, hold the barbell so your arms are bent at a 90-degree angle and your elbows are level with your shoulders.

Tip: Most people have a weaker arm – the left one if you are right-handed and vice versa. Using dumbbells instead of a barbell will help you train it to equal strength.

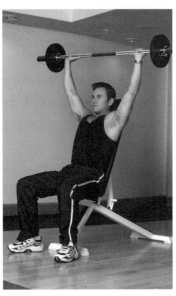

Press the bar upwards by raising your arms above your head. Hold for 1 second, then return to the start position. Keep perfect form – don't lock out your elbows (so that you keep the tension on the muscle) and make sure the weights are lowered level with your ears.

BENT-OVER ROW: 30 SECONDS

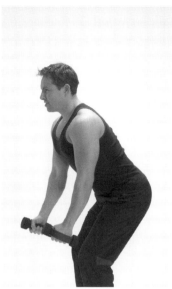

Stand with your feet shoulder-width apart, holding the weights just outside your hips. Draw your belly button back towards your spine, so your inner abdominal wall stabilizes your back. Keep knees slightly bent and bend forwards from the hips, with your abs tight and back straight. Hold the weights with straight arms, palms facing your body.

Tip: When learning any new exercise, begin with as little weight as possible. This is particularly important on this exercise, where you may suffer soreness in your lower back. In the first week, do this exercise with a broomstick, and only progress to a weighted bar when you've mastered the technique and have established that your body can deal with the lighter weights.

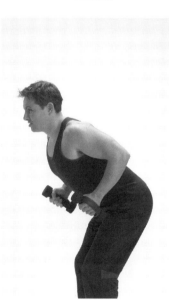

Breathing out, pull the weights up to waist level, imagining your arms are being lifted upwards and backwards by the elbows. Keep elbows pointed back – don't move them out to the sides. Finish the movement by squeezing your shoulder blades together. Hold for 2 seconds, then breathe in as you return to the start position.

DORSAL RAISES: 30 SECONDS

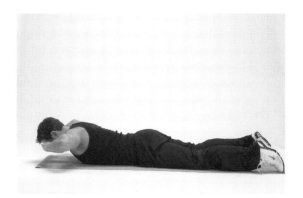

Lie on your stomach with your hands on your temples.

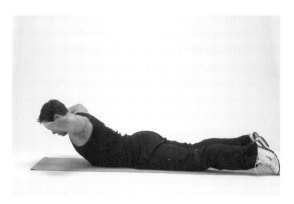

Keeping your chin tucked in, raise your upper torso off the ground without your hips leaving the floor. Lift until you feel a slight squeeze in the lower back – no higher than 6 inches (15 cm), or the point at which you can no longer maintain good form. Exhale as you lift.

Tip: To do an advanced version, lift your legs off the floor at the same time as your upper torso.

COOL-DOWN; 5 MINUTES

Skip intermittently or jog for 5 minutes, shrugging the shoulders to work out upper body tension as you allow the heart to stabilize.

STRETCH: 5 MINUTES

Do the 5-minute full-body stretch (*see* page 69).

time taken: 35 minutes

cardio workout

body benefits

Your heart, like your biceps and hamstrings, is a muscle that grows stronger with exercise. This pyramid cardio session, which involves powerwalking and running, is designed to increase dramatically your heart's pumping power and to lower your resting heart rate (a sign of fitness). You won't be able to see the effects on the inside but you will be able to feel them – you will be able to move faster, and for longer, and will have greater get-up-and-go on a daily basis. A stronger heart is more efficient at delivering oxygen to every cell in your body, leading to increased energy levels.

This workout is also a great fat-burner, burning 200–400 calories. You can tone muscles all you want but if they're still covered in excess fat no one is going to see the body beautiful underneath! When you have finished the routine, your body will fight to stabilize itself through the process of homeostasis which uses energy derived from the fat to fuel the process.

This cardio session is based on running because I find it one of the best workouts around. It works all muscles of the body simultaneously and you can do it any-where in the world, to any level. I love it for another reason as well – running gives people great thinking time. My clients find it clears the head, and banishes pent-up emotions – whether you need to laugh, cry or burn off the day's aggression, you can do it all on a run without people noticing! If you like you may swim, cycle or use a rowing machine for this session if you have good enough technique and a particular reason for wanting to do so, but, at the end of the day, I strongly advise you to run. It burns fat, tones the whole body and will get results – fast!

benefits of cardiovascular fitness

The heart is the most important muscle in the body. Here are some of the knock-on effects of greater cardiovascular fitness on your health:

- Reduced risk of heart disease and stroke;
- Lower cholesterol levels;
- Reduced blood pressure;
- Decreased body fat;
- Lower risk of diabetes.

how to pyramid train

With pyramid cardio sessions you start off walking or jogging at a comfortable pace, gradually picking it up until you reach a peak halfway through the workout, and then you gradually bring it back down again to resting. I use these sessions with clients as I find they're the most effective way to burn fat in a cardio session. Here's why:

- By peaking in the middle of a workout, rather than the end, you push at the moment where you can still extend yourself.
- Working at high intensity, even for short periods, forces the body to adapt to new levels of fitness. One of the most common mistakes people make is to do the same run 3 times a week, and wonder why a month later they aren't any fitter. You need to challenge your body, and push it to new levels, for it to grow.
- Pyramid workouts burn more calories than running at the same pace for the same amount of time. They also give a greater boost to your metabolism, so your metabolism is raised and burning more calories for up to 24 hours after the exercise session.
- They're motivating – you're going up, but you know that you're coming down. And as you gradually bring the intensity levels back down it feels like a breeze! I've found that being able to see the end in sight (any section only

lasts 150 seconds) gives people greater confidence to push themselves when it matters *and* complete the full session every time!

monitoring your rate of perceived exertion

To do a pyramid workout properly you need to monitor how hard you are working at any point in time. You could monitor the speed you are running or walking, or you could use a heart rate monitor, but in fact the most effective way to keep a track on the intensity is also the easiest – monitoring how hard the workout feels! Learning to do this makes you think about how you are feeling and it puts you in touch with your body. It also makes sure you work out to your maximum every time, without needing to waste time fiddling around with stopwatches and monitors.

To work out your personal intensity levels, use the rate of perceived exertion (PE) below. Your PE level is personal to you. Depending on your fitness levels you may reach level 9 (the ultimate challenge for your muscles and lungs) doing a very fast walk – or a sprint.

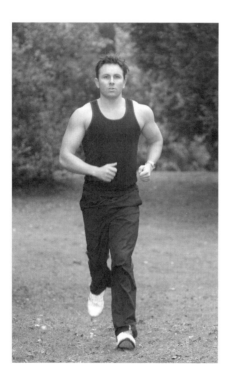

PERCEIVED EXERTION (PE)	HOW HARD DOES IT FEEL?	BREATHING	CAN YOU TALK?	% AEROBIC CAPACITY
1	Resting.	Normal.	Yes.	35
2	Minimal activity such as sitting at a desk working.	Normal.	Yes, easily.	45
3	Gentle activity – you begin to feel slightly warmer.	Comfortable.	No problem.	55
4	Your heart rate is starting to rise and you're feeling slightly warmer. Sustainable, but definitely exercise.	Deeper but regular.	Still chatting.	65
5	Quite hard. You're starting to sweat.	Deep but still steady.	Yes, but you'd rather have a conversation than do all the talking yourself!	75
6	Between hard and very hard	Getting heavier.	Still possible, but holding a conversation requires effort.	85
7	Very hard. You're sweating a lot and feeling warm.	Deep and fast.	Conversation is reduced to words rather than sentences.	90
8	Strenuous.	Very fast and deep.	One syllable.	95
9–10	The absolute hardest effort you can possibly make – you couldn't go any faster. Your muscles are burning.	Your breathing becomes laboured. You have now passed the 'anaerobic threshold'.	No.	96–100

THE PYRAMID CARDIO

The speed that you move at any time depends on your level of fitness. If you need to powerwalk at the beginning and end of the pyramid, do! And if you need to sprint up a hill at the peak of your pyramid – go for it!

Tip: Don't get stuck in a rut! Vary your running routes so you don't impose mental limits on yourself (only expecting to go a certain distance in a certain time). This will help you progress even faster.

WARM-UP: 5 MINUTES

Powerwalk or jog for 5 minutes at PE level 3.

WORKOUT: 20 MINUTES

Gradually increase the speed of your walk or running as follows:

2½ minutes at level 5
2½ minutes at level 6
2½ minutes at level 7
2½ minutes at level 8
2½ minutes at level 9
2½ minutes at level 8
2½ minutes at level 7
2½ minutes at level 6

COOL-DOWN: 5 MINUTES

Powerwalk or jog for 5 minutes at level 3

STRETCH: 5 MINUTES

Do the 5-minute full-body stretch (*see* page 69).

Tip: How fast you can go at the same rate of PE depends on your fitness and it also varies from day to day – running up the same hill can feel like level 6 one day and level 8 the next. This doesn't matter. What's important is to keep working at the same perceived intensity.

powerwalking technique

If you're just starting out on your fitness campaign you'll need to powerwalk rather than run for this workout. Powerwalking is a bit like walking as if you're 10 minutes late for a very important meeting – only with a little more technique! It places less impact on the joints than running but still puts a good cardiovascular load on the heart, and it works out the upper body. Observe good technique:

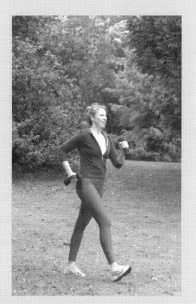

1 Hold your arms at chest level and use them in a natural rhythm – they give you momentum and help you breathe.
2 Always walk heel to toe.
3 Make sure you push off from the back leg.

As you progress, move from powerwalking to 'yomping' – interspersing very fast walking with short bursts of running.

workout time: 35 minutes

ultimate abs workouts

body benefits

These workouts will make the difference between having good abs and great abs. Although we talk about having a great six-pack, the abdominals are actually one muscle. However that doesn't mean one exercise (crunches) is all you need to train them. The secret to great abs is variation, and by doing diverse ab exercises you'll achieve a firmer, flatter, stronger midsection in less time. These exercises put emphasis on different areas of the abdominals by using different leg positions to target different abdominal fibres.

The other secret of fantastic abs is to make sure you exercise the deep stabilizing abdominal muscles, the ones that really pull in and flatten the stomach, even when you're at rest. The deep muscles are called the 'core' muscles because they compress your internal organs and straighten and strengthen the lower back. If you haven't learnt how to locate these in gym classes, practise this before you do this workout (see opposite), as your core muscles should be activated throughout all the workouts. Once they're in tone, these are the muscles that will give you great posture.

By strengthening not just your six-pack, but your entire midsection – back, front and obliques – this workout will also improve your sports performance. Your trunk is the body's central link for nearly all sports performance. External and internal obliques help you twist and bend, the deep core muscle straightens and strengthens your back. If you only work your abs, you'll get a great looking body that gets hurt as soon as you challenge it in real life or sport. That's why this workout includes lower back exercises, to keep your muscles in balance.

People's abdominal strength varies hugely, so this workout comes in two levels; beginner and advanced. The beginner's version tones abs at the same time as working to get them out from under all that abdominal fat! Start with the level that suits you: Rome wasn't built in a day, and abs can't be built in a weekend.

locating your core

Start by lying flat on your back with your legs bent at the knee and feet flat on the floor. Rock your pelvis gently so that first you flatten your spine against the floor, curling your tailbone towards the ceiling, and then release the other way. Let your spine settle in between these two extremes, in a neutral position. Exhaling, draw your stomach in from the pelvic floor upwards, thinking of trying to contract your belly button back towards your spine. Then inhale, flattening your stomach against your spine further. This is what it feels like to have your abdominals engaged. The aim is to have this active core as the starting point for all the exercises in this book.

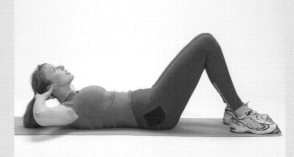

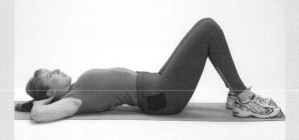

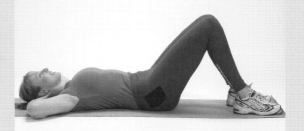

beginner ab workout

Suitable for people not currently doing any ab work, and those carrying excess body fat. Your goal is to accustom your midsection muscles to exercise and burn fat, so revealing the abs you are sculpting underneath!

WARM-UP: 2 MINUTES

Skip for 1 minute, jumping with your feet together. Spend 1 minute doing some side bends and twists to encourage blood flow to the abdominal area. This warm-up is shorter than others because with ab circuits you don't need to prepare the heart for exercise, and only need to encourage blood flow to the abdominals.

the circuit

Do 5–25 of each of the exercises below, depending on your ability. Rest for one minute and repeat (so that you complete 2 full circuits).

CRUNCHES: 1 MINUTE

These target the top section of your abdominals.

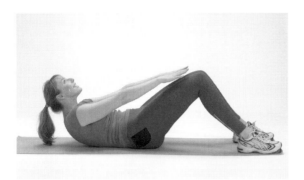

Lie on your back with your feet flat on the floor and hands on your knees. Activate your core muscles, as described above. Exhale and curl forwards, keeping your lower back on the floor and your abdominals pulled in. Keep a space the size of a fist between your chin and chest to ensure your head stays in line with your spine. Focusing your eyes on the point where the ceiling meets the wall will help keep you in alignment. Don't pull on your neck. Hold for 2 seconds. Exhale and lower.

Tip: If you get neck ache doing crunches, gently support your head in your hands. Do not curl beyond the point where you can no longer keep your abdominals flat. Remember to keep your deep abdominal muscles engaged. Do not cheat by using your hip flexors to pull you up, or using momentum from nodding your head forward.

REVERSE AB CURLS: 1 MINUTE

This targets your lower abdominals – the ones that ensure you don't have a pot belly.

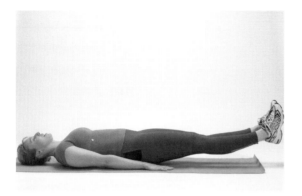

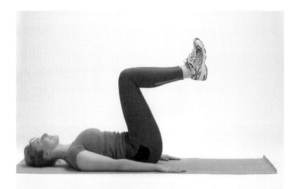

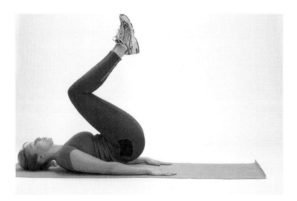

Lie flat on your back, legs outstretched and hands on the floor, palms down. Push down on palms to keep back neutral. Breathe out as you raise straight legs 6 inches (15 cm) off the floor, bend them, then breathe in as you bring knees to your chest and lift the base of your spine 3 inches (7½ cm) off the ground. Don't let your ankles touch the floor.

Tip: Hold your abdominals tight as you raise and lower your legs to protect your back. If your abs are weak you may not be able to lift your straight legs 6 inches off the floor – in which case, start and finish with legs bent and feet flat on the floor.

RAISED LEG CRUNCH: 1 MINUTE

These target the centre section of your abs.

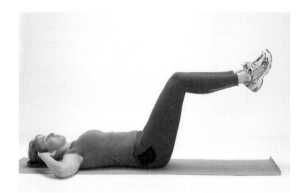

Lie on your back with your legs in the air, and your hands by your ears.

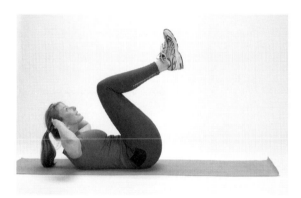

Breathe out as you bend your knees and simultaneously curl your legs towards your ribcage as you curl your shoulders forwards. Don't pull on your neck. Hold for 2 seconds, then breathe in as you return to the start position.

Tip: Keep your elbows wide and avoid pulling on your head. Ensure that you have a fist-space between your chin and chest.

SIDE TWIST: 1 MINUTE

This works your obliques to create waist definition.

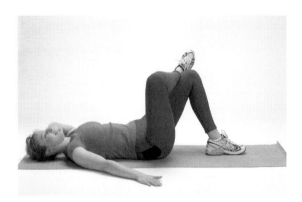

Lie back with your legs in the air. Place your right arm out at 45 degrees in the direction of movement.

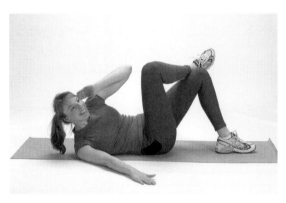

Breathe out and cross your left elbow over the opposite knee, breathe in and return to start position. Do 30 seconds on each side.

Tip: Keep abdominals tight throughout the minute.

DORSAL RAISES: 1 MINUTE

This exercise strengthens the lower back, to keep your core in balance.

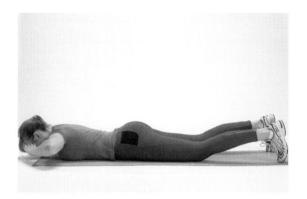

Lie on your stomach with your hands on your temples.

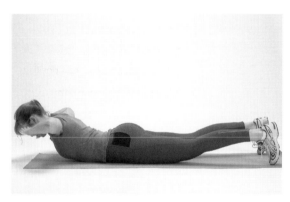

Keeping the chin tucked in, breathe out and raise your upper torso off the ground without your hips leaving the floor. Lift until you feel a slight squeeze in the lower back – no higher than 6 inches (15 cm) or the point at which you can no longer maintain good form. Breathe in and return to start position.

Tip: To do an advanced version, lift your legs off the floor at the same time as your upper torso.

pyramid run

When you have finished 2 ab circuits do a 15-minute pyramid training run, using the Perceived Exertion intensity levels described in the cardio training session (*see* page 98).

2½ minutes warm-up at level 4
2 minutes at level 5
2 minutes at level 7
2 minutes at level 9
2 minutes at level 7
2 minutes at level 5
2½ minutes cool-down at level 4

TIP: Doing the ab circuits before the run will deplete your glycogen stores before you do the run so you will burn more fat.

COOL-DOWN: 3 MINUTES

Skip or jog for 3 minutes.

STRETCH: 5 MINUTES

Complete the 5-minute full-body stretch (*see* page 69).

workout time: 37 minutes

advanced ab workout

WARM-UP: 2 MINUTES

Skip for 1 minute, jumping with your feet together. Spend 1 minute doing some side bends and twists to encourage blood flow to the abdominal area.

the circuit

Repeat the ab circuit above 4 times, with 1 minute's rest in between.

ABS: 20 MINUTES

Do 4 x 5 minute ab circuits.

COOL-DOWN: 1 MINUTE

Skip or jog for one minute.

STRETCH: 5 MINUTES

Do the 5-minute full-body stretch (*see* page 69).

workout time: 32 minutes

the plyometric circuit

body benefits

Plyometric exercises involve explosive movements that build muscle power. Cardio work and weight-training can take you only so far, but when you're looking for a way to take your body and sports performance to a new level, plyometrics are where it's at! The movements combine strength with dynamic jumps, to create explosive power and endurance, burn fat and tone the whole body. By asking the body to work out in lots of ways all at once, muscles become able to provide strength, power, balance, stamina and core stability simultaneously. Fitness is not just strength but the ability to apply strength quickly, so you have the explosive power to bounce over moguls, get off the starting blocks quickly, and play sports such as football and basketball dynamically.

Most people only attempt plyometrics when they've laid down a good base of fitness and strength through regular cardiovascular (aerobic) and weight-training. However, you can start whatever your fitness, just begin at your own pace and remember – this workout is supposed to be tough. Expect to sweat! You should feel a burn in your muscles, and your heart rate will be high throughout. The key is to keep going – failure is not an option! Only over time it will get easier. If you don't do much exercise at the moment then these sessions will be hard, but don't give in – just do as much as you can and over time your explosive power will increase.

WARM-UP: 5 MINUTES

Powerwalk, jog, skip or use a rowing or ellipsis machine for 5 minutes.

Tip: If your legs are heavy from a previous workout, do a good warm-up and stretch. This will help you feel more comfortable, by relaxing muscles and preventing injury.

THE CIRCUIT

Repeat this set of exercises 3 times, with a 1 minute rest in between sets, followed by the cool-down and stretch.

SQUAT THRUSTS (ALTERNATE LEGS): 1 MINUTE

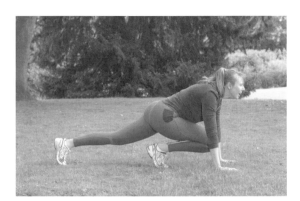

Start with your hands on the floor, shoulder-width apart, and your feet straight out behind you, in a push-up position. Bend the right leg and bring the knee up in between your arms, with your weight resting on the ball of the other foot.

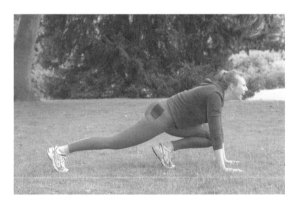

Then switch legs in a dynamic movement. Repeat as fast as possible but keeping the form. Make sure to extend the legs fully back, and keep your head and spine in alignment.

Tip: To make squats easier, place your hands on a raised static bench, in the park or gym.

BURPEES: 1 MINUTE

These are hard exercises, but they are loved by rowers for their ability to create dynamic leg power.

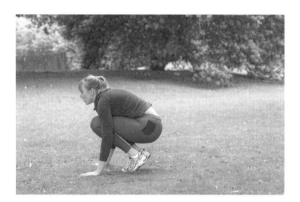

Count out an even 1-2-3-4 beat as you complete the 4-point movement.

Start by standing upright, with feet together and knees soft. Drop down to a crouch position with your hands on the floor in front of you.

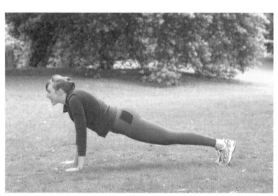

Jump your legs backwards so you end up in a full press-up position. Ensure your legs go back together at the same time.

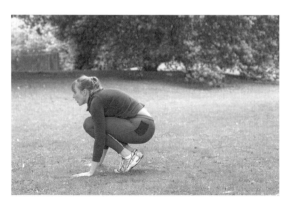

Jump your legs forwards again to the crouch position.

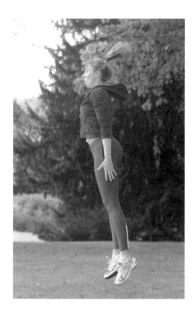

Jump up to a standing position so your feet leave the ground.

Repeat.

Tip: Stick with it, even if you need to slow down your 4-count beat. Jump as high as you can.

BENCH STEP-UPS: 1 MINUTE

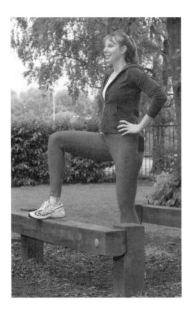

Stand facing the bench. Step up with your right foot, keeping your back straight, and placing your whole foot on the bench.

Tip: Think about pulling in your abs and curling tailbone under as you step up. Stand tall.

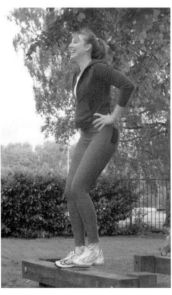

Step up with the left foot then step down, one foot at a time, right foot first. Use alternate legs to step up. If you are using stairs to do step-ups, it's fine to do two steps at a time.

SQUAT THRUSTS (BOTH LEGS): 1 MINUTE

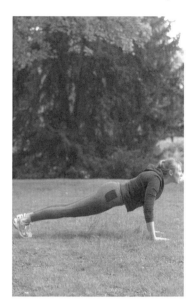

Start with hands on the floor beneath your shoulders and legs behind you, in full press-up position.

Tip: Don't compromise good form – do them properly or not at all. If need be, rest for 10 seconds and then carry on. These are the same as burpees but without the jump.

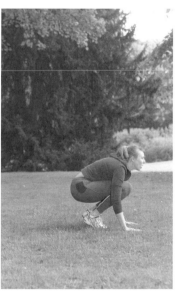

Jump your legs forwards again to the crouch position. Return to starting position, making sure to extend your legs fully back. Repeat.

SKIP: 1 MINUTE

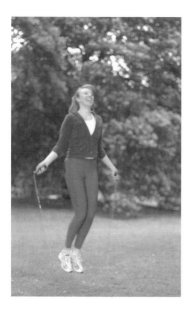

Try and skip with both feet leaving the ground at the same time, like a boxer, rather than going from one foot to the other in a running motion. It's harder but it keeps heart rate higher to burn fat and increase fitness in the shortest possible time.

COOL-DOWN: 5 MINUTES

Jog or powerwalk for 5 minutes.

STRETCH: 5 MINUTES

Do the 5-minute full-body stretch program (*see* page 69).

workout time: 33 minutes

the challenge

This is the ultimate fitness challenge. It's a one-off 50-minute test that I designed for my élite clients to do every 4 weeks as a way to track their progress. It keeps them on course and drives them on physically and mentally to succeed, giving them something to aim towards and improve on – fit people can go to the gym week in, week out, and at the end of the month face the boring realization that they've done all that work, lost no weight and are still the same shape. More encouraging if instead they can say to themselves: 'Well done, you've lost no weight and your body shape hasn't changed – but you've gained 20% more strength.' My sentiments exactly.

The idea with the Challenge is that after you've done it, you write down your results and then carry on with the program for another 4 weeks and do the Challenge again. After the first 4 weeks you might be struggling to complete the second section of the Challenge, after 8 weeks, you may not collapse till the third section – but after 12 weeks the Challenge may not be a challenge any more. Bring it on! Assess and reassess your fitness and you'll know that you're moving in the right direction and achieving your goals.

The Challenge tests you mentally and physically – can you overcome the mental blockage of doing just 1 minute of every exercise? It will test your body and mind power. Keep a positive mental attitude throughout. Just by doing this test and pushing yourself to the limit, you've already passed. Let the achievement give you self-worth. We go through our whole lives being tested emotionally, physically and mentally in some form, but you'll find what you achieve here gives you confidence and massages your ego.

If you like challenges you've probably already got butterflies in your belly just reading about what you're about to come up against. So breathe deeper, and prepare for action!

WARM-UP: 5 MINUTES

Jog, powerwalk or skip intermittently for 5 minutes till warm.

Tip: Skip on your toes, hands at hip height – both feet together for as long as possible, then alternate feet if you tire. Keep the rope tight – you need to skip quite quickly to manage this.

the circuit

Do 3 circuits of the exercises below, with 1 minutes rest in between circuits. For the first circuit, do each exercise for 1 minute. For the second circuit, do each exercise for 2 minutes. For the third circuit, do 3. Follow with the cool-down and stretch. *Remember: it's not meant to be easy!*

SQUAT THRUSTS (BOTH LEGS)

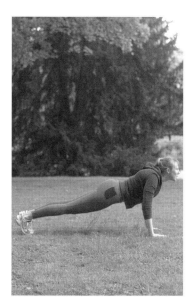

Start with your hands on the floor beneath your shoulders and legs behind you, in full press-up position.

Tip: If need be, rest for 10 seconds, then carry on. But keep pushing to challenge yourself.

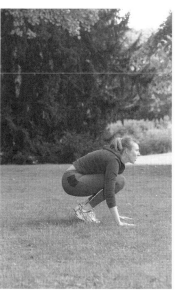

Jump your legs forwards again to the crouch position. Return to starting position, making sure to extend your legs fully back. Repeat. Don't compromise good form – do them properly or not at all.

SKIP

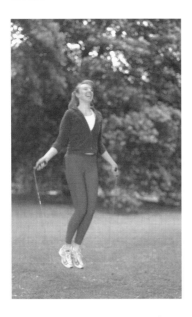

Try and skip with both feet leaving the ground at the same time, like a boxer, rather than going from one foot to the other in a running motion. It's harder but it keeps the heart rate higher to burn fat and increase fitness in the shortest possible time.

BURPEES

Count out an even 1-2-3-4 beat as you complete the 4-point movement.

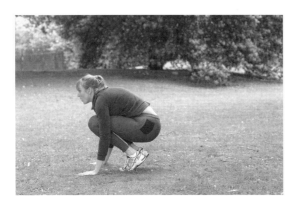

Start by standing upright, with feet together and knees soft. Drop down to a crouch position with your hands on the floor in front of you.

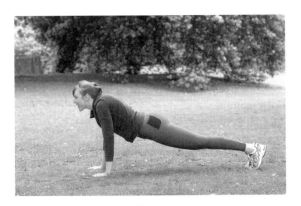

Jump your legs backwards so you end up in a full press-up position. Ensure your legs go back together at the same time.

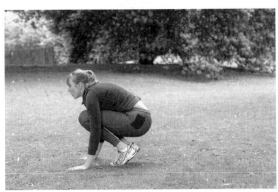

Jump your legs forwards again to the crouch position.

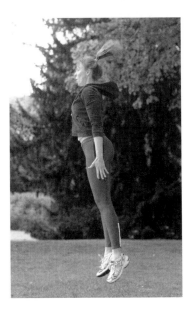

Jump up to a standing position and jump up on the spot so your feet leave the ground.

Repeat.

SKIP

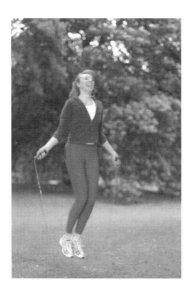

If you begin to struggle, skip intermittently.

SQUAT THRUSTS (ALTERNATE LEGS)

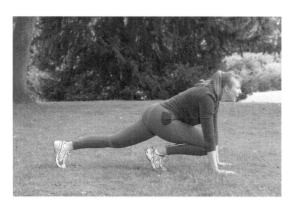

Start with your hand on the floor beneath you and your feet straight out behind you. Bend the right leg and bring the knee up in between your arms, with your weight resting on the ball of the other foot.

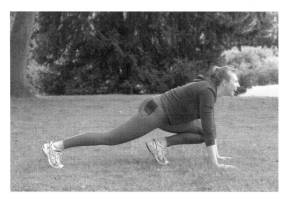

Then switch legs in a dynamic movement. Repeat as fast as possible but keep the form. Make sure to extend your legs fully back, and keep your head and spine in alignment.

SKIP

COOL-DOWN: 5 MINUTES

Powerwalk or jog for 5 minutes

STRETCH: 5 MINUTES

Do the 5-minute full-body stretch (*see* page 69).

Tip: Just remember: you're only in competition with yourself and nobody else.

workout time: 54 minutes

key points

- ■ Never workout on autopilot – pay attention to good technique and you'll get good results.
- ■ Constantly push yourself and your limits.
- ■ Never give up – it will get easier.

your body challenge exercise plan

You are now ready to test your body and resolve. This chapter contains 8 programs tailored to fit your individual aims. Each of them will push and challenge the body and mind into creating lean, defined muscle shape and strength in about just 30 minutes, 4–5 times a week. There will be moments when this will feel like the hardest thing you have ever done. But find your ideal program, stick with it, and you will come out super-fit and mentally equipped for whatever life throws at you.

You are now ready to begin the first 4 weeks of your new fitness campaign. Don't start out thinking you've got a mountain in the way – all journeys start out with a single step. Choose the program most in line with your aims, follow the exercise plan, keep your focus in the present and soon you'll be well under way – feeling fitter and stronger than ever before.

Remember: If you don't try, you'll never know how great you can be.

choosing your exercise plan

All 8 exercise plans in this book – the 7 below plus the Challenge – are hard, fast workouts that will push your body into creating lean, defined muscle shape. But depending on how you mix up the workouts, you can put the emphasis on different areas of fitness.

- **FAT LOSS** – Burns fat fast. Suitable for anyone who wants to shed excess body weight. Do this in conjunction with the fat-burning diet tips in the food chapter.
- **AB ATTACK** – A 4-week program to refine your midsection and create Geri abs. Ideal as part of your pre-summer shape up to get the ultimate beach body.
- **TOTAL TONING** – Creates a slender, leaner, more toned you, with more muscular shoulders and athletic legs. Will not bulk you up – suitable for men and women.
- **SERIOUS STRENGTH** – Will appeal to those who want to gain power, strength and definition. Use in combination with the strength-building diet tips in the food chapter.
- **SKI & TREK** – A 4-week program to create dynamic leg power and all-round fitness for the slopes. For skiers and hikers.
- **BALL SPORTS** – A mixture of strength, cardio and plyometrics work that will suit anyone playing football, hockey, rugby or any other ball sport. Will improve cardiovascular fitness and speed to the ball.
- **ACTIVE PREGNANCY** – A lighter workout for fit pregnant women.

using the diary pages

This chapter contains 4 weeks of exercise plans for each of the 8 programs, with individual tips and motivation.

There are three empty columns against each day for you to fill in. This is your book, and your program, so scribble all over it – you'll find ticking off workouts and filling in food logs is one of the easiest ways to boost your motivation. Or instead, you can photocopy the relevant pages and keep your records on them. Here's what to do in each of the columns:

COMPLETED

Put a tick against this box when you have finished your workout. If possible, fill in how many reps you did on each circuit and you will see how much you progress over time.

COMMENTS

This is the column for you to write in how you felt today. Think about your energy levels, enjoyment and overall performance. Were you tired after a hectic weekend, but still able to make a good effort? Did you feel good after a great night's sleep but a bit stiff from the day before? Make a few notes about how your workout went. If it was hard, then say so – but if you have an idea how to make it easier next time, jot that down too (did you forget to snack mid-afternoon to keep your energy up?) Always focus on the positive and use positive words, such as *'Felt tired after hectic weekend but made a good effort – and felt better afterwards.'* or *'Not used to this kind of workout so found it tough, but that means I was doing it right! Know it will help my skiing once I master it!'*

FOOD LOG

When you're trying to improve your eating habits, keeping a food log is a great way to keep yourself in check – what we think we've eaten in a day is often very different to what we've really eaten. The best way to do this is to keep a separate food log where you write down exactly what you eat and drink each day, and at what time. Write down *all* drinks, including water. And be honest – this record is for you only, so if you ate 2 packets of tortilla chips and an ice cream, then say so! In this column make notes on what was good and bad and how this linked to your performance. Did 4 cups of coffee have you buzzing by lunchtime but tired by mid-afternoon? Did you find your workout was better after eating a more substantial healthy breakfast? The key is to make suggestions to yourself on how to keep to good habits, or improve on bad ones – '*A good day until the evening – but didn't have any food at home so relied on take-out.*' or '*Drank more water and less coffee – and felt more energetic than normal!*'

MAKING CHANGES

As a personal trainer I've found that thinking can be fatal to fitness, which is why I recommend that you don't think – just follow the exercise plans that I've set out!

Trust me on this. Over the last 8 years I've toned and strengthened Halle Berry and Pierce Brosnan for Bond films, I've got Geri Halliwell fit for tours and looking fantastic, and I've helped many other people – famous and not so famous – shed up to 3 stone and revolutionize their shape from fat to fit. I've trained tennis players, footballers and marathon runners. So believe me, these plans work. The less changes you make to the plans, the fitter you'll get.

However, if something does come up – a late work meeting, a birthday party, a family obligation – you may need to do the prescribed workouts on different days to the ones suggested. If you need to switch days, abide by these rules:

- Avoid 'doubling up' sessions – the workouts are too intense to attempt to do 2 in one day, but if you feel you must, then put at least 8 hours between them (for instance, do one at 8 am, and the other after 4 pm).

- Do not do the same workout 2 days on the trot – alternating workouts (cardio on one day, lower body the next) gives your body time to recover and maximizes results.
- Never work out for more than 3 days on the trot, and always take 2–3 rest days a week. Rest is a vital part of fitness training, keeping motivation high and giving the body time to recover.
- If you really have to miss a workout, improvise. (*See* Chapter 2, 'The Mental Challenge' for ideas on how to cope with missed sessions.)

using the monthly challenge

At the end of every 4 weeks do the 50-minute Challenge to test your fitness. Write your results into the workout sheets provided to track progress. The Challenge is tough – it's meant to be – but doing it will improve your performance!

Use the progress planner (*see* page 179) to mark your progress as you go along.

frequently asked questions

How long can I stay on the Body Challenge?
Give yourself a target of 4, 8 or 12 weeks. Then give yourself a break, where you do maintenance activity or some other exercise, and then go back to it if you like. The good thing about this program is that you are doing a wide variety of different exercises, but after a while the body becomes fitness tolerant, so if you let it rest for a while and then go back to the program, you should see other benefits.

The Ab Attack and Ski & Trek plans are designed to be done for 4 weeks only, after which time you can move on to a different plan. See how you feel and listen to your body – some people work best with a routine and other people will mentally benefit from changing their plan every 4 weeks.

Can I join the workouts together for one big workout?

You can't cram fitness like you can try to cram-study. If you do 2 workouts together you won't get twice the effect. These are designed to be intense 30-minute sessions and it's impossible to keep going at that intensity for an hour.

Instead of doing a run for the cardio session, can I swim, bike or row?

I think running is the best full body cardio workout around. However if you feel you are working at the same intensity and you are being true to yourself then you can change to cycling, rowing or swimming for running in the cardio circuit. This is more appropriate for people who are strong cyclists, swimmers or rowers – if you're a weak swimmer or have never had proper rowing training, it's unlikely you'll have the technique to work out at very high intensity.

Can I do a class instead of an upper body circuit, or replace a lower body circuit with my Saturday football game?

At the end of the day you've gone out and bought this book to do the program, so you should be sticking to it as closely as possible. If you have a weekly event like squash or football, then take a rest day before it and after it and then go back to the program. The more you stick to the program, the better results you will see.

the workouts at a glance

LOWER BODY

Warm-up – 5 min

....

Squats – 1 min

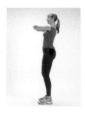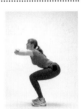

....

Alternate lunges – 30 sec each leg

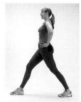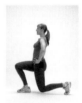

....

Sumo squats – 1 min

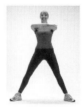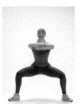

Weighted step-ups – 30 sec each leg

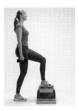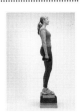

Straight-leg dead lift – 1 min

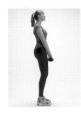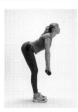

Rest – 1 min

Repeat this circuit 4 times in all

Cool-down – 5 min

Stretch – 5 min

UPPER BODY

Warm-up – 5 min

....

Press-ups on knees – 30 sec

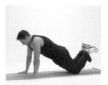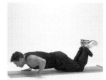

....

Full press-ups – 30 sec

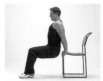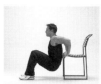

....

Pull-ups (aided) – 30 sec

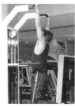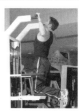

....

Tricep dips – 30 sec

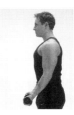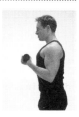

....

Bicep curls – 30 sec

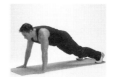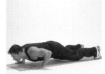

Lateral raises – 30 sec

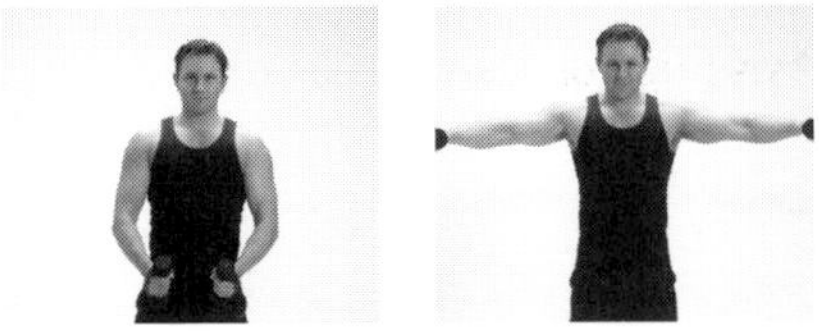

Shoulder press – 30 sec

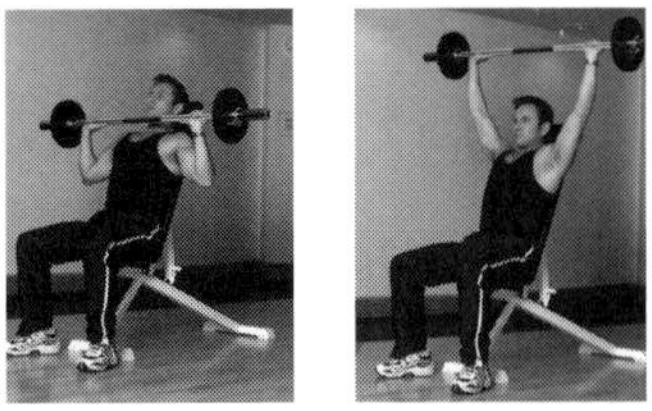

Bent-over row – 30 sec

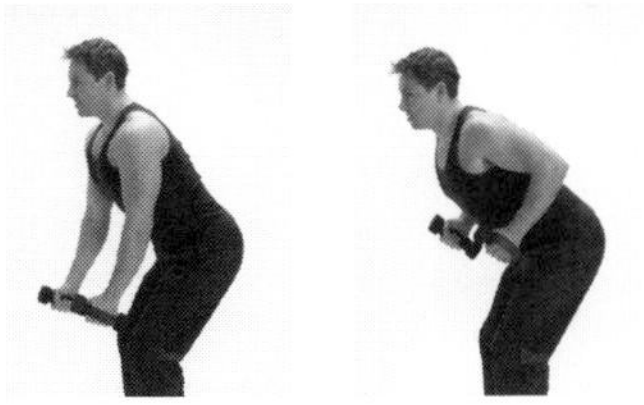

Dorsal Raises – 30 sec

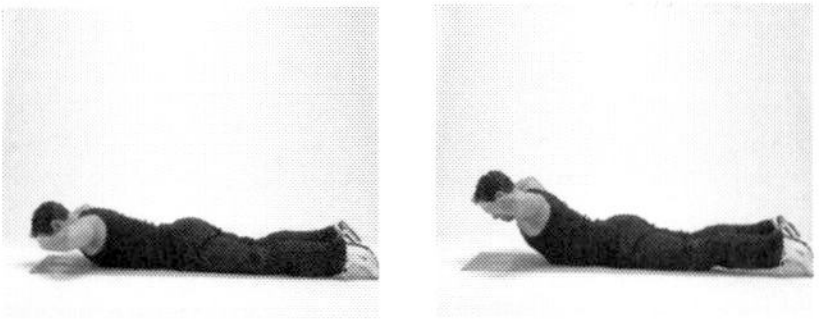

Rest – 1 min

Repeat this circuit 4 times in all

Cool-down – 5 min

Stretch – 5 min

CARDIO

Warm-up: 5 min

Pyramid workout: 20 min

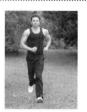 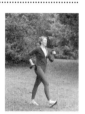

Cool-down: 5 min

Stretch: 5 min

ABDOMINALS

Warm-up – 2 min

....

Crunches – 1 min

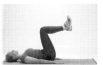

....

Reverse ab curls –
1 min

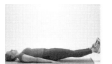 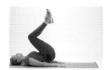 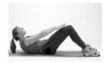

....

Raised leg crunch – 1 min

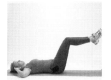 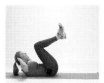

....

Side twist – 1 min

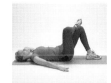 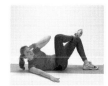

....

Dorsal raises – 1 min

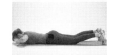 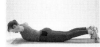

....

BEGINNER: Repeat circuit 2 times in all, then do 15-minute pyramid powerwalk or run

....

ADVANCED: Repeat circuit 4 times in all

....

Cool-down: 1 min

....

Stretch – 5 min

IMPORTANT: Pull-ups should not be attempted during pregnancy and should be omitted from the 'Active Pregnancy Program'.

PLYOMETRICS

Warm-up – 5 min

....

Squat thrust (alternate legs) – 1 min

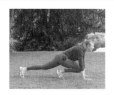 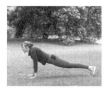

....

Burpees – 1 min

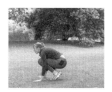 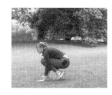

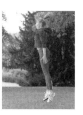

Bench step-ups – 1 min

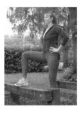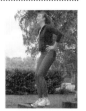

Squat thrusts (both legs) – 1 min

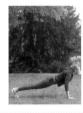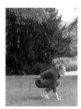

Skip – 1 min

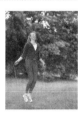

Repeat this circuit 3 times in all

Cool-down – 5 min

Stretch – 5 min

THE CHALLENGE

Warm-up: 5 min

Do 3 circuits of the exercises below.

        Circuit 1 – 1 min each exercise

        Circuit 2 – 2 min each exercise

        Circuit 3 – 3 min each exercise

Take 1 min rest between circuits.

Squat thrusts (both legs)

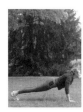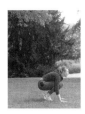

Skip

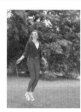

Burpees

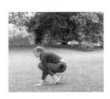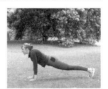

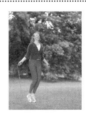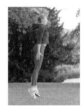

Skip

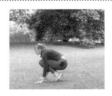

Squat thrusts (alternate legs)

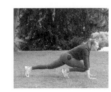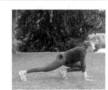

Skip

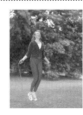

Cool-down : 5 min

Stretch: 5 min

fat loss

goal

To burn fat and lose weight, fast. These workouts burn up to 400–600 calories, and on this program people typically lose 1–3 lbs a week.

the program

5 workouts for 4 weeks. Do the Challenge on week 4, record your result, then repeat the program again. It's fine to switch some of the cardio sessions to the pool, bike or rower if you are confident enough that these will drive up your heart rate and maximize your fat burning.

Fat loss will vary from person to person. The healthiest and most efficient fat loss would be between 1–3 lbs a week for people who are 20–30 lbs over their ideal body weight, and 1–2 lbs a week for people who are between 10–20 lbs over their ideal weight. Don't try to exceed this – the body knows that fat is the most effective energy source it has, and so it wants to hold on to it. At a rate of 1–3 lbs a week the body won't notice that you're losing weight and it won't feel deprived. But if you starve yourself, your body will stop burning fat and start burning muscle instead, lowering metabolism (muscle controls metabolism) and reducing tone – exactly the opposite of what you want to achieve! This is why crash diets don't work – when you finish the diet, nice and light from shed muscle and water loss, and then start eating again, the body will put the weight back on, hence the term yo-yo dieting. Don't do it! Go in nice and slow and get results that last.

WEEK ONE

Treat yourself mean, get yourself lean. You will find this week really hard. Your brain is engaging with your body and getting it to do movements that are unnatural to you. But make a commitment to yourself: go through the learning process and do all the workouts even if you can only do 1 rep.

	WORKOUT	COMPLETED	COMMENTS	FOOD LOG
Monday	Cardio			
Tuesday	Upper Body			
Wednesday	Plyometrics			
Thursday	Rest			
Friday	Cardio			
Saturday	Lower Body			
Sunday	Rest			

WEEK TWO

New movements are now becoming engraved in your brain memory card and feeling more natural and fluent. This week won't be so hard mentally but physically you can push yourself a little bit harder. But don't go nuts — you may be keen but if you double your workout you'll overtrain! Progress gradually.

	WORKOUT	COMPLETED	COMMENTS	FOOD LOG
Monday	Abdominals			
Tuesday	Cardio			
Wednesday	Rest			
Thursday	Plyometrics			
Friday	Upper Body			
Saturday	Lower Body			
Sunday	Rest			

WEEK THREE

You will be feeling results by now. Movements will be fluent and a little bit easier, and your mental attitude will be starting to change. See yourself getting more confident in your workouts.

	WORKOUT	COMPLETED	COMMENTS	FOOD LOG
Monday	Cardio			
Tuesday	Upper Body			
Wednesday	Plyometrics			
Thursday	Rest			
Friday	Cardio			
Saturday	Lower Body			
Sunday	Rest			

WEEK FOUR

Make this your best week so far. Now you know what is contained in a month's fat-loss program, are you going to sign up for another one? Sit down and reflect on the month: what's worked, what hasn't? What can you improve on? Have you been as strict as you thought you would be at the beginning? Have you pushed yourself as hard as you thought? If you sign up for another 4 weeks, try and better what you've done: that's your challenge. (See 'The Workouts at a Glance', page 133, and Chapter 7 'The Workouts'.)

	WORKOUT	COMPLETED	COMMENTS	FOOD LOG
Monday	Abdominals			
Tuesday	Cardio			
Wednesday	Rest			
Thursday	Plyometrics			
Friday	Upper Body			
Saturday	The Challenge			
Sunday	Rest			

ab attack

goal

To create sleek strong flat abdominals. Sometimes one body part lags behind others and requires a bit more attention to catch up. This program gives you 4 weeks to get your stomach as toned as the rest of you.

program

4 workouts a week for 4 weeks. When you've finished, switch back to one of the other programs – this program is not designed to be done for more than 4 weeks.

WEEK ONE

This week is all about locating your abs and learning how to do the exercises properly. Your task is to find out where they are (if they exist!). Focus on doing the exercises properly. This is much more important than doing lots of reps.

	WORKOUT	COMPLETED	COMMENTS	FOOD LOG
Monday	Abdominals			
Tuesday	Cardio			
Wednesday	Rest			
Thursday	Cardio			
Friday	Plyometrics			
Saturday	Abdominals			
Sunday	Rest			

WEEK TWO

Now you've found your feet, get into some kind of routine mentally and try to improve your diet. The exercises should be more refined, clean and fluent than the first week, but always try to improve. Aim at being able to commandeer intense localized effort in your core muscles throughout your workouts.

	WORKOUT	COMPLETED	COMMENTS	FOOD LOG
Monday	Cardio			
Tuesday	Abdominals			
Wednesday	Plyometrics			
Thursday	Rest			
Friday	Abdominals			
Saturday	Cardio			
Sunday	Rest			

WEEK THREE

Self-evaluate and try and learn by your mistakes: are you pushing yourself hard enough? Are you focused on the job in hand? Are the exercises as clean and fluent as they could be? Don't be afraid to push yourself that extra little bit — and keep smiling.

	WORKOUT	COMPLETED	COMMENTS	FOOD LOG
Monday	Abdominals			
Tuesday	Cardio			
Wednesday	Rest			
Thursday	Cardio			
Friday	Plyometrics			
Saturday	Abdominals			
Sunday	Rest			

WEEK FOUR

By now self-esteem and confidence should be brimming and your posture should be good. Be happy at what you've achieved. It's probably not been easy on your stomach or diet, but the end is in sight! (See 'The Workouts at a Glance', page 133, and Chapter 7 'The Workouts'.)

	WORKOUT	COMPLETED	COMMENTS	FOOD LOG
Monday	Cardio			
Tuesday	Abdominals			
Wednesday	Plyometrics			
Thursday	Rest			
Friday	Abdominals			
Saturday	Cardio			
Sunday	Rest			

total toning

goal

To create lean, toned muscles all over the body. An ideal program if your body fat is quite low and you want more defined muscles.

program

5 workouts a week for 4 weeks. This program contains high amounts of resistance work together with cardio work so you can lose fat and build muscle simultaneously. Use lighter weights so you can do 20–25 reps a minute with good breathing and steady pace. After 4 weeks do the Challenge and record the results.

WEEK ONE

This week is all about location. Refine your exercises, feel every muscle in your arms, shoulders and back. Practise perfect technique.

	WORKOUT	COMPLETED	COMMENTS	FOOD LOG
Monday	Upper Body			
Tuesday	Lower Body			
Wednesday	Abdominals			
Thursday	Rest			
Friday	Plyometrics			
Saturday	Rest			
Sunday	Cardio			

WEEK TWO

Enjoy and take pride in what you are doing. Do the exercises properly. Make yourself do the workouts you hate — the exercises you start off hating you'll end up loving, once you get good at them.

	WORKOUT	COMPLETED	COMMENTS	FOOD LOG
Monday	Upper Body			
Tuesday	Abdominals			
Wednesday	Rest			
Thursday	Lower Body			
Friday	Cardio			
Saturday	Plyometrics			
Sunday	Rest			

WEEK THREE

By this time you should be starting to feel like you're gaining tone. The exercises will start to seem easier and flow a lot quicker but remember to keep perfect form.

	WORKOUT	COMPLETED	COMMENTS	FOOD LOG
Monday	Upper Body			
Tuesday	Lower Body			
Wednesday	Abdominals			
Thursday	Rest			
Friday	Plyometrics			
Saturday	Rest			
Sunday	Cardio			

WEEK FOUR

This is the final week, so maintain focus and drive. Concentrate! Ensure you have a good week and remember you have the test (the Challenge) at the end of it. (See 'The Workouts at a Glance', page 133, and Chapter 7 'The Workouts'.)

	WORKOUT	COMPLETED	COMMENTS	FOOD LOG
Monday	Upper Body			
Tuesday	Abdominals			
Wednesday	Rest			
Thursday	Lower Body			
Friday	Cardio			
Saturday	The Challenge			
Sunday	Rest			

serious strength

goal

To build muscles and strength. Ideal for those looking to turn their bodies into a powerhouse.

program

5 workouts a week for 4 weeks. Use heavier weights, so you can do 8–10 reps in a minute, using slow controlled movements. Increase weights used gradually over the weeks, but never compromise technique for a heavier weight. On the Saturday of every Week 4 do the Challenge. This is an ideal program to repeat for up to 12 weeks.

WEEK ONE

Get to know your body. People who are training for a bit more strength need to locate the right muscle groups for an exercise. Get to know what weight you have to lift to get to 8–10 reps.

	WORKOUT	COMPLETED	COMMENTS	FOOD LOG
Monday	Upper Body			
Tuesday	Lower Body			
Wednesday	Abdominals			
Thursday	Rest			
Friday	Plyometrics			
Saturday	Upper Body			
Sunday	Rest			

WEEK TWO

Strength is one of those things where you have to train with a little bit of aggression sometimes — but don't substitute aggression for form. Strength comes from moving muscles correctly. Make sure you're not cheating by getting other muscles to do the work (such as using small body thrusts to help you do curls, rather than standing still and isolating your bicep alone).

	WORKOUT	COMPLETED	COMMENTS	FOOD LOG
Monday	Lower Body			
Tuesday	Abdominals			
Wednesday	Upper Body			
Thursday	Rest			
Friday	Plyometrics			
Saturday	Lower Body			
Sunday	Rest			

WEEK THREE

Your body should be starting to feel a little bit stronger, and the exercises will become a little bit easier so put the weights up if you feel you can. Time to add a few more kilos, but don't sacrifice form. Don't train your ego, train your body — it doesn't matter if you're lifting less than someone else in the gym, if you are lifting it well. Make sure people are staring at you for the right reasons (your form) not the wrong reasons (your weight is too heavy and your technique is rubbish!)

	WORKOUT	COMPLETED	COMMENTS	FOOD LOG
Monday	Upper Body			
Tuesday	Lower Body			
Wednesday	Abdominals			
Thursday	Rest			
Friday	Plyometrics			
Saturday	Upper Body			
Sunday	Rest			

WEEK FOUR

You should be on top form. Motivation will be running high, and you'll be training on a lot of adrenalin, aggression and explosive strength. Your body should be feeling as if it's tightening and strengthening. Ensure you maintain correct breathing and form and put the weights up a bit – strength is an aspect of fitness that increases quickly when trained. (See 'The Workouts at a Glance', page 133, and Chapter 7 'The Workouts'.)

	WORKOUT	COMPLETED	COMMENTS	FOOD LOG
Monday	Lower Body			
Tuesday	Abdominals			
Wednesday	Upper Body			
Thursday	Rest			
Friday	Plyometrics			
Saturday	Lower Body			
Sunday	Rest			

ski and trek

goal

To build explosive leg power to bounce over moguls, climb up hills, and have the endurance to hike or ski all day.

program

This is a 4-week program to help you get in shape for skiing and hiking holidays. It builds a well-balanced body, dynamic power in the legs, and strength in the heart. It's designed to be done for 4 weeks before a skiing holiday, but if you want to start training in advance of that, do the fat-loss or toning program. You don't need to do the Challenge at the end of it – by the 28th day you should be on the flight ready for your holiday! If you are a snowboarder, switch one or two of the upper body sessions to an ab circuit.

WEEK ONE

Your skiing holiday is 4 weeks away. Don't worry if you are aching a little bit at the end of this week — you'll be fully recovered by the time your holiday comes around.

	WORKOUT	COMPLETED	COMMENTS	FOOD LOG
Monday	Plyometrics			
Tuesday	Rest			
Wednesday	Lower Body			
Thursday	Cardio			
Friday	Upper Body			
Saturday	Rest			
Sunday	Lower Body			

WEEK TWO

Focus on the positive: you're going to improve your skiing or hiking by doing this. Right now you'll be sore, but your body is refining and adjusting itself, so you can ski more dynamically.

	WORKOUT	COMPLETED	COMMENTS	FOOD LOG
Monday	Plyometrics			
Tuesday	Upper Body			
Wednesday	Rest			
Thursday	Lower Body			
Friday	Cardio			
Saturday	Abdominals			
Sunday	Rest			

WEEK THREE

Hopefully this program will allow you to ski longer, faster and harder. Keep going and you'll be able to graduate from red runs to black runs, and from black runs to off-piste.

	WORKOUT	COMPLETED	COMMENTS	FOOD LOG
Monday	Plyometrics			
Tuesday	Rest			
Wednesday	Lower Body			
Thursday	Cardio			
Friday	Upper Body			
Saturday	Rest			
Sunday	Lower Body			

WEEK FOUR

You should be brimming with confidence, and have belief in your body's ability to ski at a higher level. Your body is now strong, toned and ready for anything that the piste can offer you. Good luck, ski well! (See 'The Workouts at a Glance', page 133, and Chapter 7 'The Workouts'.)

	WORKOUT	COMPLETED	COMMENTS	FOOD LOG
Monday	Plyometrics			
Tuesday	Upper Body			
Wednesday	Rest			
Thursday	Lower Body			
Friday	Cardio			
Saturday	Abdominals			
Sunday	Rest			

ball sports

goal

To improve your speed to the ball and your endurance on the pitch. Football, hockey, rugby and other ball sports all require dynamic balance, fitness and leg power for short springs.

program

5 workouts a week for 4 weeks. If you're playing a game, that counts as a workout. Drop one of the workouts and adjust the program so you take a rest day before match day.

This program builds fast and slow twitch muscle fibres so you have endurance and explosive speed.

WEEK ONE

Remember, by working out you're actually improving your ball sports, not hindering it. You're allowing the body to become more dynamic with greater strength, endurance and stamina.

	WORKOUT	COMPLETED	COMMENTS	FOOD LOG
Monday	Upper Body			
Tuesday	Lower Body			
Wednesday	Cardio			
Thursday	Rest			
Friday	Abdominals			
Saturday	Plyometrics			
Sunday	Rest			

WEEK TWO

The fitness you are gaining will prolong your ball-sport career and give you the edge over players who haven't both-
ered to do pre-season fitness training. Keep going — you'll be sharper both mentally and physically.

	WORKOUT	COMPLETED	COMMENTS	FOOD LOG
Monday	Upper Body			
Tuesday	Lower Body			
Wednesday	Cardio			
Thursday	Rest			
Friday	Abdominals			
Saturday	Plyometrics			
Sunday	Rest			

WEEK THREE

With ball sports, practice makes perfect, so do some ball work as well as body work this week. Use the energy tips in the diet chapter to make sure you have usable fuel on match days.

	WORKOUT	COMPLETED	COMMENTS	FOOD LOG
Monday	Upper Body			
Tuesday	Lower Body			
Wednesday	Cardio			
Thursday	Rest			
Friday	Abdominals			
Saturday	Plyometrics			
Sunday	Rest			

WEEK FOUR

By doing this program you are being injury preventative. Stick with it – it's going to allow the body to adapt to knocks, help you ride tackles, and help prevent problems in your ankles, shins and knees. (See 'The Workouts at a Glance', page 133, and Chapter 7 'The Workouts'.)

	WORKOUT	COMPLETED	COMMENTS	FOOD LOG
Monday	Upper Body			
Tuesday	Lower Body			
Wednesday	Cardio			
Thursday	Rest			
Friday	Abdominals			
Saturday	Plyometrics			
Sunday	Rest			

active pregnancy

goal

To maintain a healthy heart for you and your baby. This program is only for continuing exercises for women who are fit pre-pregnancy – never start a program like this when you're pregnant and unfit. This is a time to keep up some light safe maintenance exercise for a happy, healthy pregnancy, but not to start anything new.

program

5 workouts a week for as many weeks as you like during your pregnancy. Unlike the other programs this is a suggestion, not a prescription. When you're pregnant, the most important thing you can do is listen to your body and work within its limits. Keep safety in mind:

- Make sure you consult your doctor or physician before embarking on any fitness program. If you have any symptoms of discomfort then consult your doctor.
- Start gently – use light weights and low reps.
- Preferably powerwalk rather than jog.
- When you are pregnant it is not recommended that you lift weights above shoulder height. Pull-ups are therefore omitted from the upper body workout.
- There will become a point in your pregnancy where press-ups on the floor become difficult, at which point graduate to a bench.
- Listen to your body – only do the exercises that feel comfortable.

WEEK ONE

Don't think because you're pregnant that you have to be sedentary. I've trained women right up until they've given birth — one client had a session on the day she gave birth! Pregnancy actually gives women a lot of energy in certain months, and you can use this for fitness. Just do what feels comfortable.

	WORKOUT	COMPLETED	COMMENTS	FOOD LOG
Monday	Cardio			
Tuesday	Upper Body (excluding pull-ups)			
Wednesday	Rest			
Thursday	Lower Body			
Friday	Cardio			
Saturday	Upper Body (excluding pull-ups)			
Sunday	Rest			

WEEK TWO

Remember that you're not eating for two – it's more like one and a bit!

	WORKOUT	COMPLETED	COMMENTS	FOOD LOG
Monday	Lower Body			
Tuesday	Cardio			
Wednesday	Rest			
Thursday	Upper Body (excluding pull-ups)			
Friday	Cardio			
Saturday	Rest			
Sunday	Lower Body			

WEEK THREE

Use pregnancy as your motivation this week – being fit makes things easier when you've had your baby. Not only do you get back in shape quicker, but you'll have more energy for your baby. And when you're in labour you'll find it easier to push.

	WORKOUT	COMPLETED	COMMENTS	FOOD LOG
Monday	Cardio			
Tuesday	Upper Body (excluding pull-ups)			
Wednesday	Rest			
Thursday	Lower Body			
Friday	Cardio			
Saturday	Upper Body (excluding pull-ups)			
Sunday	Rest			

WEEK FOUR

Remember that people find pregnant women beautiful and blossoming. You don't have to feel that you are fat and over-weight, there is such a thing as fit pregnancy! (See 'The Workouts at a Glance', page 133, and Chapter 7 'The Workouts'.)

	WORKOUT	COMPLETED	COMMENTS	FOOD LOG
Monday	Lower Body			
Tuesday	Cardio			
Wednesday	Rest			
Thursday	Upper Body (excluding pull-ups)			
Friday	Cardio			
Saturday	Rest			
Sunday	Lower Body			

the body challenge progress planner

The Challenge is meant to be difficult – what is the point of easy challenges! Use this page to chart your progress on the Challenge and see how you match up to the goals you have set yourself. Remember, you can't fail the Challenge – just attempting it is a sign of a well-tuned mental attitude and a level of physical fitness that is prepared to give it a go. We all have our good and bad days, so try and do the Challenge when you are feeling 100%.

DATE	RESULTS

the way forwards

All these workouts are designed to be mixed and matched. Knowledge is power and now you have the knowledge to create your own workouts it is up to you to use it. Keep empowering yourself by creating and designing for yourself fresh workout variations based on the sound principles set out in this book. Constantly set yourself new challenges and, always, keep moving forwards. Good Luck!

resources

UK

Fitness Industry Association (UK)
115 Eastbourne Mews
Paddington
London W2 6LQ

Tel: 020 7298 6730
Fax: 020 7298 6731
E-mail: info@fia.org.uk
Website: www.fia.org.uk

British Journal of Sports Medicine
BMJ Publishing Group
BMA House
Tavistock Square
London WC1H 9JR

Website: sss.bjsm.bmjjournals.com

USA

American Council on Exercise (ACE)
4851 Paramount Drive
San Diego
CA 92123

Tel: (858) 279 8227; (800) 825 3636
Fax: (858) 279 8064
Website: www.acefitness.com

American College of Sports Medicine
401 W. Michigan Street
Indianapolis
IN 46202 3233

Tel: (317) 637 9200
Fax: (317) 634 7817
Website: www.acsm.org

Commando Workout

Simon Waterson

4 WEEKS TO TOTAL FITNESS

Commando regiments are the fitness elite of the modern military. Their mantra is *Improvise, Adapt and Overcome*. Often training without the luxury of a gym, the commandos have developed a workout system that builds fitness fast and is completely adaptable.

Now you too can experience the challenges and rewards this dramatically effective training program offers.

- Prepare your mind first so your body will follow
- 30-minute workouts for quick results
- Burn calories through the day after your morning workout
- Special outdoor and gym workouts
- How an exercise buddy will keep you motivated
- Adaptable exercises tailored to your lifestyle
- Techniques to develop upper and lower body definition
- Effective fat-burning, stamina-building nutrition plan

the ultimate personal training kit

This unique 'fit kit' is your own personal trainer. As the military take essential kit with them everywhere they go, the Simon Waterson Ultimate Personal Training Kit holds basic fitness and workout items that can be used in a variety of different ways. Designed to be taken on holiday, to the office, or to the park, it is perfect for those who want to take their workout wherever they go.

This stylish, compact backpack contains:

- Interchangeable dumbbells
- Skipping rope
- Resistance band with handles
- Dynoband
- Stopwatch
- Waterbottle
- Sweatband and neck towel
- Specially designed workout cards designed by Simon Waterson

A fantastic gift for anyone about to embark on an exercise plan or for anyone who takes their personal fitness seriously, the Ultimate Personal Training Kit can be ordered from my website: www.simonwaterson.com

Thank you, keep fit and, most of all, have fun!

Make
www.thorsonselement.com
your online sanctuary

Get online information, inspiration and
guidance to help you on the path to physical
and spiritual well-being. Drawing on the integrity
and vision of our authors and titles, and with
health advice, articles, astrology, tarot, a
meditation zone, author interviews and events
listings, www.thorsonselement.com is a great
alternative to help create space and peace
in our lives.

So if you've always wondered about practising
yoga, following an allergy-free diet, using the
tarot or getting a life coach, we can point you
in the right direction.

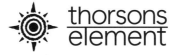

thorsons
element